To Rich!

Thank you for it
Your flow with me it
the Hacienda Del Sol Resort
in Tucson! You are a
pleasure ♡ Danielle

Testimonies

"Danielle has been able to address all levels of health and motivation in our International Corporation. We have experienced tremendous, sustainable results over the years like significant weight loss, reduction in prescription drug use, better morality and increased productivity in our company."

-Richard Lively, VP Human Resources, Clinton, New Jersey

"Danielle asks the hard questions that direct change.
Get ready to question your self-perception and body confidence."

Anne Mankiewich, Personal Trainer, South Harpswell, Maine

"Her work gave me simple and flexible tools that took the guesswork out of managing a healthy lifestyle change."

Chris Turner-Noteware, City Director, Dallas, Texas

"She has a way of getting people (even their pets) involved in a healthy and active lifestyle."

Sheree Mueller, Business Owner, Rainbow City, Alabama

Until you heal the wounds of your past, you're going to bleed. You can bandage the bleeding with food, alcohol, drugs, work, cigarettes, shopping and sex, but eventually, your pain will ooze through and stain your life. You must find the strength to open the wounds, stick your hands inside, pull out the core of your pain that's holding you in your past, and make peace with the memories.

-Iyanla Vanzant

Evolve Healthy®

A Mindfulness Guide for Food & Body Liberation

Jacquelin Danielle, RDN, CSCS

Evolve Healthy®

A Mindfulness Guide for Food & Body Liberation

Jacquelin Danielle, RDN, CSCS

Contact Danielle for book signings, workshops, seminars, retreats and speaking events:

MindfulBodyRevolution.com

Social Media

Facebook: JacquelinDanielleRD
Instagram: JacquelinDanielle
LinkedIN: JacquelinDanielle
YouTube: JacquelinDanielle

Book Cover Design: Hok Michael Hawkins - MindCanvas.com
Food Dairy Design: Kevin Johnson
Editors: April Jones, Olivia Kendrick
Photographers: Janet Moran-Lankford,
Bekki Parker Lawson, Michael Harvey

First Edition - Printed in the USA

River
Songbird
Publishing

Dedication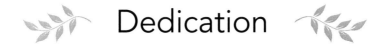

I dedicate this book to the minds that bully their own bodies;
for those that hunger for self awareness, mind expansion and body liberation.

My prayer: That choosing to utilize these steps guides your path
towards falling in love...*with you.*

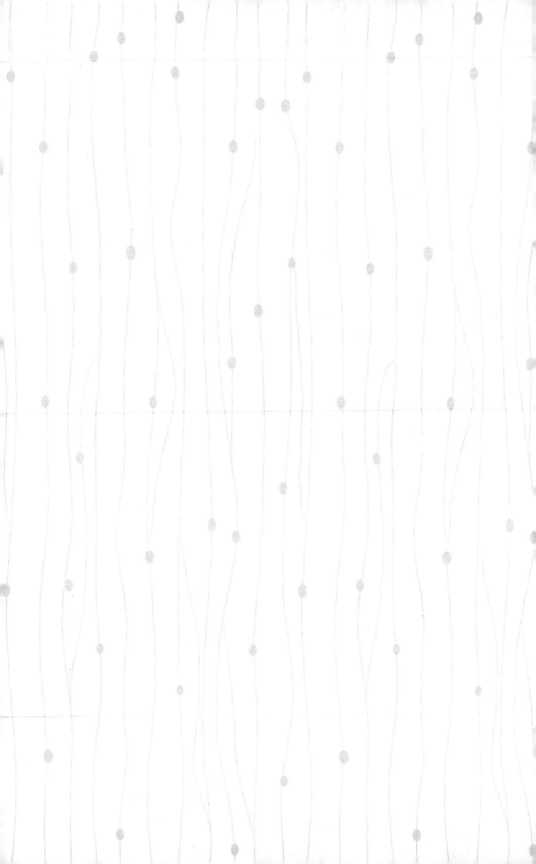

Table of Contents

We ask ourselves, Who am I to be brilliant, gorgeous, talented, fabulous? Actually, who are you not to be? You are a child of God. Your playing small does not serve the world."

-Marianne Williamson

Introduction

Evolve Healthy is a lifestyle guide rooted in spirituality and science. This seven-phased system will support positive behavior changes specific to: nutrition, exercise, sleep, body confidence and stress management. *Evolve Healthy* will inspire you to shift your perceptions and ideas of "healthy" while aiding the liberation of your well-being. Guided personal assessments will help you acknowledge and address limiting behaviors that have a stronghold on your happiness. Finally, a practical nutrition plan that will help you improve your diet by using basic food journaling techniques to boost body awareness and halt emotional eating. No more tracking calories, and grams to lose weight-it's time you revolutionize your relationship with food and your body!

_____ *Do you feel guilty or ashamed when you eat unhealthy foods?*

_____ *Are you an emotional eater?*

_____ *Do you wish you had more energy to be more active?*

_____ *Do you have difficulty getting a good night's sleep?*

_____ *Do you feel your body is not good enough no matter how much or how little you invest into it?*

If you answered 'yes' to one or more of these questions, you're in good company.

Evolve Healthy® includes:

(1) *Personal Assessments*: Train the mind to embody a healthy lifestyle behaviors. Practice shifting your thoughts and recognizing your emotions. These actions will empower healthier choices.

(2) *Practical Nutrition Plans*: Learn sustainable meal planning and food preparation strategies. Train your senses to stimulate food satisfaction and enhance food choice quality, quantity and balance.

(3) *Intentional Movement*: Practice moving with activity or exercise that celebrates life. Choose a type that works for you--motion is lotion for the body.

(4) *Good Sleep Education*: Honor the importance of sleep. Develop an ideal bedtime ritual that changes your life!

(5) *Sweet Spot*: Achieve body confidence by practicing self-love; know your worth NOW, not waiting until "_____" happens first.

(6) *Stress Management Strategies*: Learn what outlets work best for you by practicing release options. One size never fits all!

I am not fully healed,
I am not fully wise,
I am still on my way.
What matters is that I am moving forward.

-Yung Pueblo

Embrace the glorious mess that you are.

-Elizabeth Gilbert

‹ My Story ›

At one point, my physical body was a burden and an obsession. Beginning at the age of thirteen, and continuing into adulthood, I told myself I was not enough. The voice varied, depending on what area was under scrutiny: not tall, or short enough; not big, or strong enough; not lean, or small enough. Regardless of where I looked, the story was always the same, "I am not enough." I was NEVER "enough". I suffered in my inability to be grateful for my body for many years. My distorted body image was thereafter accompanied with disordered eating. Through many seasons, I could not believe my body was perfectly made by my Creator.

Like many of us, I grew up inside a dysfunctional family. It included alchohol abuse, co-dependency, and schizophrenia. I was the middle child who felt the need to *save* my family. I was hurt and angry, but mostly, I wanted to be perfect. Journals have long been a way for me to process, release and discern. As an adult, I discovered an entry from the age of fifteen that read, "If I am perfect, I will ease these painful emotions inside me. If I can ease the emotions inside of me, I will surely make them proud and ease their pain too."

My first food binge was an entire box of strawberry breakfast bars. Home alone after school, I can recall how sweet the taste of that one, small bar (oh, how I craved sweetness in my life!). I decided to eat another…then another…until the box was empty. Afterward, a cloud of shame and guilt concealed me. I grabbed the box with its empty wrappers and shoved them deep into the trash. I would tell no one that I had lost control. I would tell no one that I was not perfect. I did not want to be judged or be called attention hungry, but I was. I needed to be seen; to know that I mattered. After multiple crazy eating episodes, I knew my thinking was off. I didn't like the idea that food had taken control of me, but I wanted to learn how I could justify what I ate and still rock a great body.

Therefore, I declared war and committed myself to learning the art of food manipulation! I decided to become educated (and ultimately heal myself). With knowledge, I could dictate how, when, where and why food was going to work for me! I began reading every nutrition article I could get my hands on. There I was, eating and reading; realizing the way I was eating was not optimal as an athlete (gymnast). I read tons of magazines in high school and then talked to my peers about the information I was learning. Their reaction? Surprise and confusion. I was small and didn't have a weight problem. They were disgusted with me and told me I had an eating disorder. I was defensive and in denial. I thought they were big because they seemed so much bigger than me, and I was terrified to be as big as them. In my mind, to be the best gymnast I could be, I had to be small-especially if I wanted to go on to college gymnastics. Looking back, they were not big, and I was tiny.

I kept reading about nutrition through high school and college. The hypocrisy of food and nutrition confused me because all the information I was reading was so contradictory (1993-1997). During an appointment with my college advisor, I realized I wanted to be a dietitian. I had to know the truth about food! I was food and body obsessed and looking for my education to cure me.

By that time, I was starting to fill out and I wanted to fill out in the "right" places: butt, legs, sculpted abs— you get the picture. The girls in fitness magazines became my ideal picture of self. In 1999, I started entering fitness competitions, and I quickly took note at my first one that I was a twig in comparison. I was surrounded by muscular women. All of a sudden, instead of eating less, I had to start eating more to gain muscle. So, I began the frightening process of eating more food, more often.

While this had initially irritated me, it was a catalyst for shifting my mind from food deprivation to muscular growth. As I became educated in dietetics, I realized that food was not the root of my suffering. My torment was deeper than the food itself. Food was a way for me to escape my emotions. When I ate less, I felt in charge.

When I ate more, it was because I hungered for comfort, companionship and sedation. I was at war against myself in the battlefield of my own mind. With an intentional search for understanding, I knew it was going to take more than education to heal, so I sought help at the University Student Center. Involved with therapy for the remaining years of college, I consulted with a psychologist who specialized in eating disorders. I remember singing some of the lyrics to her which so strongly resonated with me at the time from "Foolish Games" by Jewel, "…these foolish games are tearing me apart". To me, this song was about wearing a mask, and my mask was perfection and control.

> *When I ate less, I felt in charge. When I ate more, I hungered for comfort, companionship and sedation. I was at war against myself in the battle-field of my own mind.*

After I graduated with a dietetics degree, I did not share my story. I was fearful that people would judge me as a recovering food addict, and unable to hear me as an educated professional. I kept it a secret. It wasn't until a divine appointment empowered me to share my raw truths to others facing the same trials. My first experience was while working, fresh out of college, as a dietitian. A teenage girl came into the nutrition clinic. She was struggling with body acceptance, restricting and binge eating. I knew she was angry and sad. Because of my own journey, I could meet her where she was without trying to fix her emotions. I watched her eyes fill with hope as I shared my eating disorder story. It was the first time I could *truly see,* with my soul, how powerful it was to share my secret with another human being. The authenticity of my struggle, and the fragmented process of my recovery is what comforted her-not my degree or job title. I grew to realize I didn't have to be a perfect, know-it-all professional to help others. I just had to speak from my heart and meet people where they were, including myself.

I'm now forty two years old and most minutes of the day, I'm at peace with my body. I've done a lot of inner work to get here. Although, I am keenly aware that I am not done. I have more to my evolution. Everyday I must *choose* to practice the mindset of changing what I can and accepting what I cannot. My intention is to continue uncovering my strongholds, so that I might be liberated from them! That I might be a role model for the generations after me who bully their bodies like I have. Not despite the fact I struggle, but because I struggle. I know that I am going to be okay; that I am not alone. It helps me to remember that my body was not meant to last; it is temporary instrument to experience my humanity; here and gone in a flash. The aging process is real and I must *choose* to age gracefully. I must *choose* to remember food is to fuel, nourish and heal me, and it can be enjoyed. The gift of my body was not for obsession or enslavement. **My revolution:** I will share my story of radical healing and conscious action. I will tend to my mind, body and soul, so that it may bring love, empathy, creativity, passion, and well-being into this world.

Dear one, this book will challenge you to tend to your physcial, emotional and spiritual well-being. I believe you are ready for this, or you would not read this far. Note: This book is not for the weak hearted. It involves shadow work and self reflection during moments of reactivity. It will ask you to *notice* (not fix) both positive and negative emotions and where they live inside your body. Sometimes it hurts. Upon completion of these seven phases, especially with an accountability partner or small group, *you will be different.* I invite you to embody a journey of radical healing and conscious action. Take a deep breath through your nose and let it out your mouth. Turn the page. Your evolution continues...

Namaste,

Jacquelin Danielle

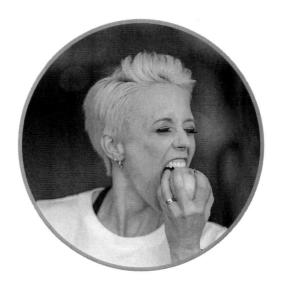

How to Evolve Healthy®

Each phase of this book includes personal assessments to evolve your mindset, body awareness, and relationship with food. You may choose to journey the seven-phased system alone or with others. Partners or small groups are encouraged to meet once a week for fellowship and accountability.

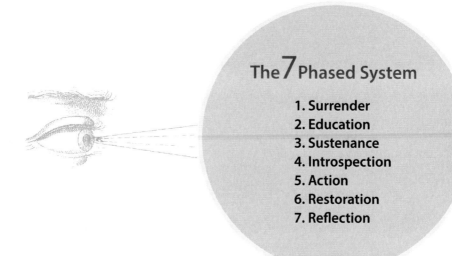

The 7 Phased System

1. Surrender
2. Education
3. Sustenance
4. Introspection
5. Action
6. Restoration
7. Reflection

What to expect:

- Seven phases completed in 7-14 weeks. It is your choice to complete one phase per week, or one phase every two weeks.

- Work alone, with a partner, or in a small group (a small group is between 3-20 participants). This program may be completed alone, however there is often great healing and power found in having accountability when processing pain with others. If working with others, schedule your weekly meetings in advance. One book per participant will be needed.

- Personal assessments. There are several personal assessments in each phase intended to enhance mental clarity, discernment and focus.

- Sweet Spot. These *play dates* are invitations that encourage healthy lifestyle practices and boost self-estem.

- Food journal each day using the *Evolve Healthy*® Food Diary, located in the back of this book. Each time you consume food or beverage you will record three specifics:
  1. Food and beverage sources (i.e. almonds, water).
  2. Clock time (i.e. 2pm).
  3. Emotion(s) you are experiencing (i.e. angry, sad).

The ultimate goal of this nutrition plan is to *create awareness*. By tracking food choices, meal timing and the emotions present, you can begin to observe and reveal behavior patterns. For example: "I am feeling anxious and in need of something sweet". In this example, discovering a repeated food entry may reveal a need for comfort when anxious. To heal you must be willing to feel it in your body while simultaneously observing your mind. This allows the space required to unlearn unhealthy behaviors and rewrite your body chemistry. For some, it may be advisable to work through this with a life coach or licensed counselor, as some of this may elicit a deeper emotional response than anticipated.

There's more than one answer to these questions pointing me in a crooked line.
And the less I seek my source for some definitive, the closer I am to fine.

-Indigo Girls, Closer to Fine

Phase I: Surrender

Do you feel guilty after eating unhealthy foods because you want to be healthy and lose weight? This opening phase defines the importance of food behavior awareness and the thoughts attached to the behaviors.

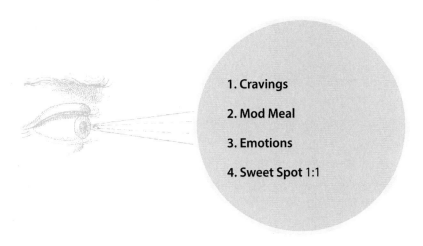

1. Cravings

2. Mod Meal

3. Emotions

4. Sweet Spot 1:1

CRAVINGS

There is a collective knowledge about what to eat and how to exercise, but our behaviors are often counter intuitive. Why is it that we temporarily harness self-discipline, eat nutritious foods, begin exercise programs, lose excess body weight, and feel great only to return to the body composition we worked so hard to transform? Old patterns are rich in comfort and difficult to change. When we are willing to expose the comfort connections to the violations we have allowed, we can move more swiftly toward change.

Subconsciously, commitments can be completely opposite of those we say we have. For example, you may say, "I am committed to losing weight". However, you find yourself eating unhealthy foods later that same day or within a few days of committing to this choice. Instead, the subconscious commitment *must be* " I will live my life spontaneously and do what I want to do." To evolve behaviors, we must expose, own, then practice a method that empowers sustainable lifestyle changes.

The world teaches us to judge and hide our mistakes, remain attached to outcomes, and resist cravings completely-this *is not* practical. What IS practical is the decision to pay attention to our mistakes, our attachments and our cravings as they arise. This is a mindfulness practice. The good news is there is no finish line and the practice will never cease to be less than interesting. As we pay attention to our behaviors, we can opt in or out of changing them. This improves our ability to determine why...and what... we find ourselves craving in the first place. For example, the moment we realize that our food choice is a poor one, we have made a conscious observation. The inner dialogue might go like this, "I know I should not eat this, but..." In that very moment, instead of dismissing the call of your craving to act out, ask yourself, **"What am I really craving?"** If you can be honest and answer this question, you are on the path! Any exposure is the journey to food freedom. Sometimes, the same exposure can be revealed multiple times in one day. Hallelujah! Every time you expose it and surrender it, you are choosing to heal; another layer of the real you is being revealed.

What are you really craving?

?

What do you need to surrender?

Personal Assessment 1:1

Let us ask in prayer, for our hearts to be searched, and our thoughts, behaviors, and mind-made stories be revealed. These stories have us turning to food as a source of comfort. The goal of this assignment is to surrender your cravings, witness your thoughts and move through them.

We eat for a myriad of reasons. We use food to escape or validate emotions, to fuel our bodies, and to celebrate. Some of us eat because it is tasty and we like to experience flavor. Eating is a necessary practice and it is to be celebrated and enjoyed. Understanding why and what we eat can help us create more informed choices. To consider why we eat what we choose creates clarity, and clarity makes room for change.

Complete this assignment while you are sitting still with your eyes closed, or taking a walk. Ask from the deepest center of yourself, **"Why do I eat?"** and, **"Why do I choose that type of food?"** As thoughts arise, sit with whatever may surface for as much time as you can. Be patient and gentle with yourself. Document your observation. There is no pass or fail to this assessment. With awareness, you will begin to understand why you have specific food cravings.

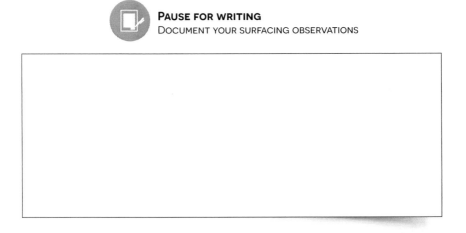

PAUSE FOR WRITING
DOCUMENT YOUR SURFACING OBSERVATIONS

Mod Meals

Mod is short for the word modification. The word modification means to "temper, soften, adjust, alter, change, refine or revise modifying something." [1] Conscious, moderated, unhealthy food splurges are not the enemy. This acronym does not have to stand for "Meal of Death"! Mod Meals are experiences that do not have to take us over. Unhealthy foods may be incorporated into your weekly Mod Meal. REMEMBER... I said, Mod MEAL, not Mod DAY, y'all! The nutrition plan includes a once a week, prescheduled, Mod Meal. As mindful eating patterns evolve, you may not feel the urge to indulge every week. That's okay! But if you are spontaneously indulging and feeling guilty about it, then you may find it beneficial to add a once a week Mod Meal into your meal plan.

Without boundaries, we fall back into our unconscious thinking, which is the opposite of mindfulness. Unconscious thinking has consequences.

Mod Meals have boundaries much like a sport has rules, a business has standard operating procedures, or a child has parameters on where to play. Without boundaries, we fall back into our unconscious thinking, which is the opposite of mindfulness. Unconscious thinking has consequences. To say that you can never eat unhealthy foods again would be very challenging and unsustainable in our culture. When we create too much restriction, the mind often forms ideas of self-sabotage. A benefit of the Mod Meal is that it grants permission to experience unhealthy foods while serving as a weekly reminder that eating healthy feels better. This proactive approach invites all food types to be enjoyed without the judgmental mind static. Practicing a Mod Meal will cultivate awareness and self-discipline.

Research Professor and Author Brene Brown stated, "Shame needs three things to grow exponentially in our lives: secrecy, silence, and judgment." [2] Therefore, permission to live this Mod Meal out loud and enjoy every single moment of it! **What foods do you enjoy the most?**

Personal Assessment 1:2

Time to encourage your food cravings and discover your Mod Meal food favorites! Holy yum! What foods do you crave? Below is a framework for you to work through. There are boundaries around this assignment. Healthy boundaries are important in any relationship, including your relationship with food. First, consider this question carefully, maybe even reading it aloud:

What are my favorite unhealthy foods

I often crave and sometimes overeat?

It's okay to give yourself some time to contemplate your answers. Choose foods and beverages that you desire to experience on a weekly basis. Not necessarily ALL of them each week, but if you had to narrow it down, what would the list look like? For example, my favorite unhealthy choices are burgers and ice cream. Mostly, it's the nostalgia of them. They were comfort foods for me when I was a child. For me, these unhealthy indulgences are worth having every week. Maybe yours is not quite as unhealthy as mine; perhaps you prefer to overeat a healthier choice, such as a big serving of mashed potatoes with butter. My unhealthy food list used to be a long mental list. However, when asked myself the same question, my extensive mental list became three written items. My list has become shorter over time and so may yours. It's okay if your list is longer. In time, you may discover there are only a few items that make the written cut.

List your favorite unhealthy foods below. Remember, these are the foods you'll enjoy at your your weekly Mod Meal.

PAUSE FOR WRITING
DOCUMENT YOUR SURFACING OBSERVATIONS

Are you an emotional eater? My observation is that we all are. Why wouldn't we be? Humans have emotions all day long and the body must eat. Emotions are bodily sensations that we feel through the middle of our body—from the base of our spine to the crown of our head. Emotions are the response to what we are thinking. Emotions are how the subconscious mind communicates what we find important. It is said that there are seven human emotions: [3]

Fear • Lust • Anger • Pride • Courage • Acceptance • Peace

Of course, there are other emotions that fall within these seven categories; love, mad, glad, sad, happy, scared, confused and bored, just to name a few. When we are experiencing an emotion, it is an enlightening experience to ask, **"Where do I feel this in my body?"** You can answer the question if you first allow yourself to feel the emotion. Pay attention. Notice the body sensations that live inside your body's emotional centers. These esoteric traditions of Indian religions, new age medicine, and psychology are know as the chakras.

The emotional centers and their meaning are denoted with a slash, as each emotional center hosts the spectrum of opposites, yin and yang.

1. Base of the spine (root)—Fear/Trust
2. At the navel (sacral)—Lust/Creativity
3. 2-3 inches above the Navel (solar plexus)—Anger/Power
4. Center of chest at the sternum (heart)—Pride/Love
5. Base of the throat (throat)—Courage/Communication
6. Between the eyes (third eye)—Acceptance/Awareness
7. Top & above the head (crown)—Peace/Spirituality

Personal Assessment 1:3

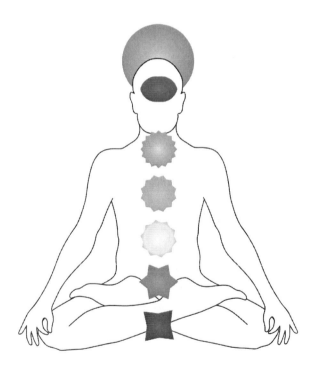

*There is an abundance of information available on chakra energy centers. If this topic interests you, I encourage you to do some personal research on this specific topic. It is a vast topic that is worth learning and understanding.

Mindful eating is the practice of observation, awareness, releasing judgment and presence amidst consumption. [4] When we are present, we savor, relish the taste, chew more slowly and digest food more effectively. Mindful eating cultivates new eating behaviors, because you can more clearly sense the body's cues that tell you when to eat and stop eating. [5] Whether the food is healthy or unhealthy is not the point. The point of mindful eating is to change your relationship with food entirely. Mindful eating can change the way you think on a cellular level. Rather than reacting to a thought that urges you to overeat or restrict, you respond to the thought without allowing it to take over. Healthier ways to cope with thoughts will be practiced throughout this curriculum, such as mindful breathing and meditation. With diligent practice, you may realize you no longer manage your emotions with food. You can learn to tolerate your uncomfortable emotions without pushing them away or stuffing them down with food.

Let's practice!

Choose a food item you would like to experience. It can be a berry, a piece of chocolate, a cracker, whatever you want! Go get that food item right now. I'll wait right here…

Now, **before** you take the first bite, bring your attention to your emotional status and answer the following questions.

What am I feeling right now?

Where do I feel this in my body?

- Now, take a deep breath all the way down to your hips.

- Go ahead and take a small bite.

- Close your eyes, chew and swallow. Listen and observe.

- Document any observations, experiences or thoughts.

PAUSE FOR WRITING
DOCUMENT YOUR SURFACING OBSERVATIONS

Mod Meals

Triggers are uncomfortable *emotions* that arise from inside of you: anger, anxiety, frustration, jealousy, and abandonment, to list a few. Triggers are direct links to our emotional wounds; wounds that were created from painful life experiences. Triggers are like built in antennas rooted by an unpleasant emotional memory. When we ignore or choose not to accept certain emotions, as painful as they may be, the emotions go into hiding from our mind and fester inside our body. We can be quite trigger happy, without any certainty of why. Oftentimes, we are unsure in which experience the roots lie. However, if we do some self-inquiry, we can uncover the origin of these roots. The body has an intelligence far beyond its anatomy. It has a story that needs to be told. Listening to your body does not require fixing it, but instead, it allows the opprotunity for you to meet it with greater understanding so the tension may be released. If you can understand this concept, eventually you will move toward gratitude when you notice a trigger. For example, when someone makes me feel angry, I can say to myself, "Damn, that's a trigger!" Then, if I am willing to inquire, because I desire to heal the wounded story, I may ask myself, **"What is this trigger asking me to heal?"**

I used food to escape my emotional pain. I began the hunt for my next food fix as soon as my big emotions were brimming. I didn't know what to do with them. For a long time, I was not aware that this was what was happening. My emotional eating would occur when I was not physically hungry, and usually soon after I was triggered. As I grew into this awareness, I slowed down. Little by little, the evolution occurred.

What you choose to eat is not as important as asking yourself the questions before you respond to the emotion. **"What am I feeling right now and where do I feel it in my body?"** Sometimes, new awareness can be difficult to digest. Often, we become fearful of what is bubbling up to the surface. We freeze, retreat and turn back to old, safe patterns. Consider the following acronyms. I developed these to help me move past fear.

C.A.R.E.

C. *CHANGE IT*. Can you change it? (Remember, you *cannot* change other people). Yes? Great. Take the next step to cultivate change. No? (Go to **A**.)

A. *ACCEPT IT*. Can you accept it? Yes? Great. Take the next step to cultivate acceptance. No? (Go to **R**.)

R. *REMOVE YOURSELF*. When you can not change nor accept something or someone, you may choose to remove yourself from it/them. Is this a necessary step? Yes? Okay. Take the next step to remove yourself. No? (Return to **C**.)

E. *EVOLVE*. Whether you chose **C. A.** or **R**. you will evolve. Taking initiative to drive your **C.A.R**. is to move you along in your human experience with greater awareness.

J.A.R.

When you find yourself in an emotional battle or an environment that has you feeling uneasy, ask yourself, "**Am I putting myself into a J.A.R.?**" We often place ourselves in a **JAR** when we are missing the mark. **J**udgement, **A**ttachment and **R**esistance keep us from experiencing freedom in every moment. Be present and gentle with yourself when you realize this.

J. *JUDGEMENT*. Who or what are you judging? Can you stop and C.A.R.E.?

A. *ATTACHMENT*. Who or what outcome are you attached to? Can you stop and C.A.R.E.?

R. *RESISTANCE*. Who or what outcome are you resisting? Can you stop and C.A.R.E.?

S SWEET SPOT

Sweet Spots are built into this curriculum to encourage playful and creative development. For you Type A personalities like myself, it's always a good time to practice flowing through life in the grey area; taking life *a bit* less seriously!

Over the years while practicing nutrition therapy, people often say to me, "I need something sweet every day," to which I inquire, **"What is sweet in your life right now?"** The question quiets most people. In that pause, I ask, **"Are you getting enough sweetness in your life right now?"** At that point, they either look at me like a deer in headlights or their eyes tear up. I then ask, **"Are you turning to food for sweetness because you need more sweetness in your life?"**

Sugary edibles will rarely satisfy your sweet spot for very long. Yet, throughout this book, you can expect to find these sweet endeavours. These activities will help guide you back to understanding that food cannot fill all your cravings. These Sweet Spots will help realign your food behaviors and mindset, by giving you ideas for self care. These hands on experiences are like "icing on the cake", with each Phase being the cake. Think of these Sweet Spots like an emotional buffet, where you can come back for seconds! The sweetest part: it's not cheating and you won't gain weight!

S SWEET SPOT 1:1

It is time to experience your first Mod Meal, mindfully. Think about what favorite foods and environment you would you like to experience this week. Plan the date and go! Experience the event with attention: tasting each bite, being present with your food, feeling what your body is expressing before, during and after you eat; feeling the emotion attached to this experience or this food choice. (i.e. guilt, regret, pleasure or joy.) What does your food choice bring to mind (fear, beliefs, myths, or memories)? Eat and be mindful! Afterward, journal your experience.

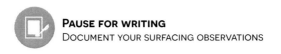

PAUSE FOR WRITING
DOCUMENT YOUR SURFACING OBSERVATIONS

References

1. Modification. Merriam-Webster website. http://www.merriamwebster.com/dictionary/modification. Accessed March 25, 2018.

2. Brene Brown on *Shame: It cannot survive empathy.* http://www.huffingtonpost.com/2013/08/26 brene-brown-shame. Accessed January 3, 2017.

3. Our Seven Life Force Energy Centers. http://www.expressionsofspirit.com/yoga/chakras.html. Accessed January 12, 2017

4. Mindfulness. Merriam-Webster website. http://www.merriamwebster.com/dictionary/mindfulness. Accessed March 25, 2018.

5. Kabat-Zinn, J. *Coming to Our Senses: Healing Ourselves and the World Through Mindfulness.* 1st ed. New York, NY: Hyperion; 2005.

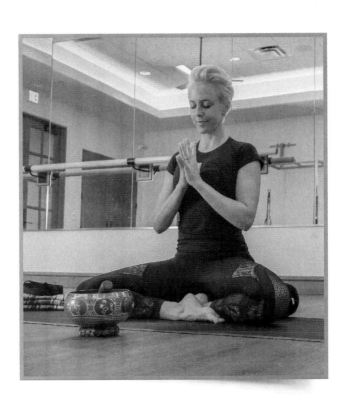

*W*ork your mind and the body will follow.

-Byron Katie

Phase II: Education

In this phase, you will learn how to choose nourishing foods with simple preparation techniques and basic food grouping. The education phase will explain the relationship between food and the body. Learn sustainable nutrition plans and food preparation strategies while training your senses to enhance food choice.

1. Proactive Plan
2. Sweet Spot 2:1
3. Nutrition
      - Clean Eating
      - Macronutrients
      - Carbohydrates
      - Dirty Dozen & Clean Fifteen
      - Acceptable Processed Food
      - Sodium
      - Alcohol

Part 1: Proactive Plan

Strategic planning reminds us of where we are going and what we need to get there. The core framework for success is to establish direction and create realistic goals. Proactive is the opposite of reactive. With proactive planning, your health goals have an empowered direction instead of becoming a victim of circumstance.

There are fifteen Proactive Plan worksheets in the index of this book.

Complete one proactive plan each week.

I like to complete my Proactive Plan on Sunday's. Choose any day of the week that works for you! Pick it and stick to it. Try to be consistent with that same day throughout the program. Each week, I encourage you to plan for five specific things. You will write these down on the proactive plan worksheet using a pencil! Divine Wisdom sometimes laughs at our hard nosed plans. Writing in pencil allows for unexpected, but necessary changes. With that said, upon initially writing your plan, have full intention to do it! If something becomes a barrier to your commitment, and you have PEACE about changing the plan, erase and rewrite it for another day. Do your best to reschedule it within the same week. If you notice you are consistently rescheduling, notice what is taking precedence in your life right now. It's not about if it's good or bad, simply NOTICE what is important.

Five things to plan each week:

1. Movement (150-360 minutes/week)

Intentional movement is also known as a workout, exercise, fitness, activity, etc. It is any kind of movement that you do (on purpose) to increase your normal heart rate and keep it there. This is called a steady state cardiovascular zone. Being intentional about choices can provide movement that celebrates life! It is important that you enjoy the way you move for health benefits. If you despise going to the gym, don't go to the gym! If you like walking outside with your dog, do that! There is a plethora of movement options. We just have to ask ourselves, **"What do I like doing, and am I willing to do it?"**

Each week, write down the exercise type, and the time (in minutes) it will take to perform each session.

Slice up your 150-360 minutes each week however works best for you. You may want to enjoy two, 10-20 minute sessions each day. Or, you may like moving for 30 minutes most days, with a 60-minute session during the weekend. Each week may be different; that's why completing a weekly Proactive Plan is helpful.

Choose a movement that inspires you in a setting that is convenient to the flow of your life. Also, consider a space that provides refuge. This will help you identify it as an outlet, not a chore. You can move in your home, outdoors, at the gym, or other facilities. Here are a few of my personal favorites that are convenient to the flow of my life right now: dancing in my living room, yoga on my patio, or at a nearby studio, strength training at home or the gym, hiking, walking my dog, and qi gong in my back yard. Having a list of my favorites helps to recognize what activities I can make time for, on a regular basis.

How do you like to move? If it's been awhile since you've exercised-I've got you! Please take the step and get into your body! It's a decision that you will never regret. Now is the time to begin again. If need be, start slow and steady and build up from there. Be realistic and true to yourself. **What can you see yourself doing this week for intentional movement?**

Grab your pencil! Document **two ways** you will move with intention this week (i.e. walk my dog every day for ten minutes, ride my bicycle around the block three times, dance in the living room for twenty minutes a day, go to the gym three times a week).

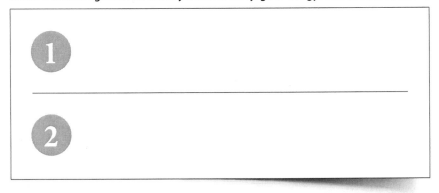

Personal Assessment 2:1

As your stamina increases, your list of ways to exercise may increase too. As a backup or goal list for other ways to exercise, **what are some other FAVORITE ways to move?** (i.e. roller skating, cycling, mountain biking, stand up paddle board (SUP), rock climbing, line dancing) Depending on where you live, family schedules, etc., some things may require greater effort on your part to include each week.

Document two additional ways you can make time for movement:

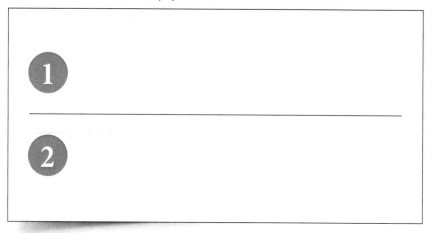

2. Food Shop

Each week, write down which day you will food shop. Much like a scheduled workout, hair appointment or party date, we set a date for it and make it a priority! Planning a specific day to grocery shop or visit the farmer's market is vital to making healthy food choices. The decision to shop once a week rather than haphazardly will simplify your life and decrease your mental stress. No more, saying, "Ah, I'm out of fruit today! I guess I'll have to eat these chips instead." When we restock the cupboards, refrigerator and freezer with healthy foods we will be equipped to eat them.

3. Meal Prep

Each week, write down the day to prepare food for the week. Adding a meal prep hour (or two) to your weekly schedule takes the guesswork out of meal planning. Meal prepping has many benefits. Here are a few:

- Helps control portion sizes
- Allows packing food on the go
- Helps you choose (and eat) healthy, balanced meals
- Stops you from being tempted by unhealthy foods
- Allows you to save money once spent on fast food
- Saves you time out of the kitchen

Personally, I do not love cooking. I want food to fuel my body and taste good, but mostly, I want it to be ready when I am hungry; especially while on the go. It is best to schedule your meal prep within 24 hours of your food shopping. Consider all the foods that take time to prepare and make them a part of your meal prep power hour! If you do not like leftovers, I must warn you—it can be more challenging to eat healthy without a weekly meal prep. I'm not saying it cannot be done, but I encourage you to change your mind about leftover food. Althernatively, you could invest in your local meal prep company. Preferrably one that prepares balanced, wholesome, and fresh meals. Bottom line—making time to meal prep each week can make your food choices easier!

Here are some of my favorite examples of meal prepping:

- Washing, slicing and chopping vegetables in advance. This makes it one step easier to come home from work and cook your veggies.
- Preparing additional quantities and cooking for more than one meal at a time. Last night's healthy dinner makes for tomorrow's lunch or dinner too!
- Washing fruit in advance for grabbing on the go.

- Pre-make smoothies and freeze for grab and go options.
- Make homemade hummus that lasts all week in the fridge.
- Boil seven or more eggs. Cooked eggs last seven days in the refrigerator.
- Line up "on-the-go" containers or baggies and drop a shot glass (1.5 ounces) full of almonds and raisins. This makes for many quick "grab-and-go" unprocessed snacks.
- Cook a pot of brown rice as a quick base for many meals.
- Cook oatmeal with nuts and dried fruit and reheat for breakfast.
- Grill an entire pack of poultry to deduct an hour of cooking each day.
- Bake several whole yams.
- Assemble meals in containers for the week with frozen vegetables, lean proteins, and whole grains.

4. Mod Meal

Each week, write down the day your Mod Meal will occur. (You established your favorite Mod Meal food choices in personal assessment 1:2, page 19.) When scheduling your once a week Mod Meal, consider your upcoming week. Do you have any obligatory meetings, social events, or other circumstances that offer foods you want to eat? Perhaps, but you don't want to worry about what foods to choose in this setting. For example:

Party time!
You are going to a social event that is serving food.
Lunch meetings!
If you have a catered meeting and you have no idea what will be served.
Date night!
Who wants to eat healthy when they eat out? Not me! I want to eat what I want when I dine out, because I only dine out once a week.
Just because!
You get to stretch your food boundaries once a week! Think about what it is that you REALLY want—treat yourself to just that! (This is my favorite. It's 100% personal choice in celebrating your Mod Meal favorite foods!)

Healthy meals require organization and demand foresight. Be prepared (pack and carry lunches to work; have snacks while your kids are playing sports; while traveling all day on an airplane, etc.). The good news is food shopping and food prep take away most of the struggle to eat healthy on the go.

5. Self-care

Each week, plan a day for "S"elf-care! Self, with a capital "S" is specific to nourishing your higher Self. Our souls are comprised of thoughts, emotions, choices and will. Through Self-care we find new inspiration, restoration and playful energy. Are you giving yourself permission to nourish, tend to, and replenish YOU? How about on a weekly basis? Some of you may already practice Self-care! If so, keep it up! Most people are so immersed in the daily grind that they forget to plan some time for themselves to soothe, recharge and contemplate what is happening in their lives. Over the years, I have learned to make time for this yummy treat. It has facilitated growth in my confidence to trust and love on myself. I have marveled watching my clients evolve their self-compassion, self-respect, and self-love with this effort! It may feel ackward at first, but hang on. You will soon realize that Self-care is essential, potent ingredient to feel healthy.

A Self-care appointment doesn't have to be active, but of course, it can be if that is what feels nourishing to you. I invite you to go on this date with yourself. You may prefer others to be present, however, Self-care is an opportunity to explore, wonder and become receptive to new energy arising from the experience. Many people abandon the things they like to do when getting involved in a relationship; oftentimes, because their 'other' doesn't engage in the same things. Shame and guilt sneak their way into your head and you may stop making time for the things that nurture your soul. When we expect only the company of others to fill our need for fun, we limit ourselves from hearing our own inner voice. Community and relationships are wonderful for the human spirit. It is nice to come together and experience one another. Nonetheless, going on a date with yourself is empowering, inspirational, and enlightening. You may even be inspired to evolve this once a week date to an annual vacation. Here are a few collective favorites of Self-care activities:

- **Go to a movie**
- **Go to the theatre**
- **Go see a concert**
- **Paddle on the water**
- **Take a bubble bath**
- **Paint or draw**
- **Write**
- **Journal**
- **Doodle**
- **Nap**
- **Read**
- **Go on a road trip**
- **Play music**
- **Listen to music**
- **Go out to dinner**
- **Take a hike**
- **Take lessons**
- **Get a massage**
- **Enjoy a salon visit**
- **Go to a workshop**
- **Go to a retreat**
- **Meditate**
- **Yoga Nidra**
- **Do arts and crafts**
- **Go to a sport outing or event**
- **Bowl**
- **Camp**

PAUSE FOR WRITING

WRITE DOWN OTHER SELF-CARE ACTIVITES THAT COME TO MIND

Personal Assessment 2:2

Describe your ideal day.

PAUSE FOR WRITING
BE AS EXAGGERATIVE AS POSSIBLE

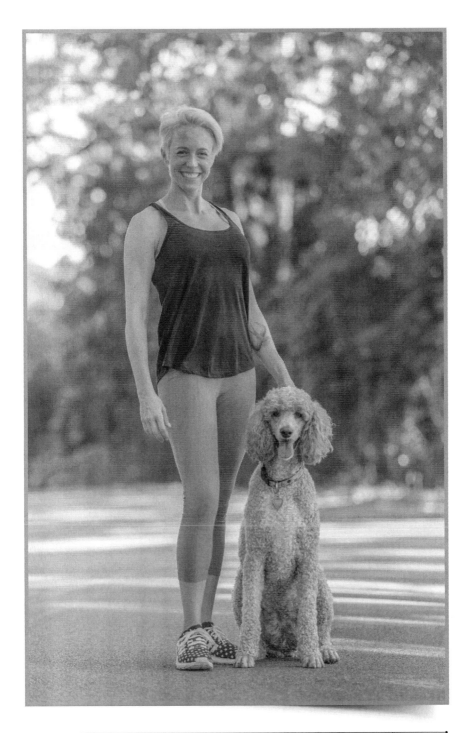

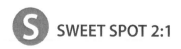

Have you ever taken yourself out on a date? When is the last time you did something by yourself, because *you wanted to go,* but no one was able to accompany you? This Sweet Spot will be an act of courage for many. I know it was for me. When I do courageous things for myself, by myself, my self-confidence increases in a way I can literally feel down into my bones. TOWANDA! One of my personal mottos for courage is, "Feel the fear, and do it anyway!" Prepare your mind to contemplate this scenario. What would you do? Where would you go? What would this look like ventured alone? For me, going on a cross country road trip by myself seemed like a liberating thought for years. I never would do it, because I was afraid to go alone. Then, I drove 2,000 miles in four days from Alabama to Arizona. It was an incredible experience that I will never want to forget. Another time, I went to see The Indigo Girls in concert. I was gifted a ticket by complete strangers, while waiting in line at the box office. This Divine compensation, is one of my favorite memories. This Sweet Spot exercise is a delicious opprotunity to experience the greatest love of your life...YOU!

Part 2: Food & Nutrition

It has become evident that billions of dollars are being made from confusing the masses about food. In twenty years of my professional work as a registered dietitian-nutritionist, I have observed this misunderstanding and intentional disinformation at the expense of people's wellbeing. The trendy and ever evolving food fad diets, buzzwords, gimmicks and "quick fixes" are heavily marketed. If we don't know any better, we may buy into them because we want to feel and look better. The issue is, most of what is being pitched is unsustainable. Everything works for the first two weeks, but then what? Our media and food industry provide a misrepresentation of what it means to be "healthy". [1]

I have highlighted seven "somewhat confusing" nutrition words currently being used by food manufacturers that address scientific aspects which are, more often than not, misleading for consumers.

1. Clean Eating

It is said that clean foods had a mother, grew from the ground (blossomed from a plant or tree) and you can pronounce all the ingredients. Most foods today are fortified and enriched with vitamins and minerals to improve nutrition quality. Enrichment and fortification began in the first half of the 20th century when diets in the United States consisted of a limited number of foods that were produced on local farms. When people have only a few foods available to eat for a long period of time, they are likely to develop a vitamin or mineral deficiency. By adding nutrients to commonly eaten foods, such as corn meal and flour, many nutrient deficiencies in the US became extremely rare. Today, we have an amazing variety of foods we can enjoy daily so we do not have the nutrient deficiencies that were common one hundred years ago. Some fortified foods help address current public health problems, such as the addition of folic acid (a B vitamin) to grains, which prevents birth defects. Although, we need some fortification for the general public, I will confess that I do love the original clean eating concept that originated within the body building community decades ago. Clean eating is a call to action for understanding the transparency of food. Fundamentally, it is a good message that says, "Let's get back to the basics with whole food and include a variety of foods in all food groups." Clean foods like whole grains, fruits, non-starchy and starchy vegetables, nuts, seeds, butter, coconut oil, legumes, dairy, eggs, meat, fish, and poultry provide nutritional balance. The original concept did not imply that there is a "dirty" or non hygienic way of eating compared to "clean eating". However, that interpretation has occurred with the commercialization of clean eating it in the past decade. As with most food fads, the commercially driven aspect of clean eating made healthy eating confusing.

The original concept is to eat less processed and more fresh food! While it may be true that most of us cannot sustain a lifestyle of clean eating, while being exposed to American food culture, especially if you enjoy dining out on a regular basis. Yet, it is wise to be mindful of what foods are considered nonprocessed, enhanced, overly processed, or downright junk. Whether you embrace clean eating or not, it is important to realize that non processed foods have significant value as food medicine. Whenever you consume fast food and overly processed foods that contain LARGE amounts of artificial ingredients, additives, or preservatives, your body suffers.

The consequences of making poor food choices are astounding. America has never been more obese than it is right now. The Trust for America's Health projects that forty-four percent of Americans will be obese by 2030 while the Centers for Disease Control and Prevention projects forty-two percent of adults. [2] The American Heart Association (AHA) reports that twenty-three percent of adults currently have metabolic syndrome. [3] Metabolic syndrome is related to obesity and this epidemic is on the rise. The five risk factors that increase the likelihood of developing metabolic syndrome, including heart disease, diabetes and stroke are:

1. **Increased blood pressure**
2. **High blood sugar levels (insulin resistance)**
3. **Central obesity (belly fat)**
4. **High triglycerides**
5. **Low levels of good cholesterol (HDL)**

Because processed foods contain too much sugar and saturated fat, and too little dietary fiber, eating less of them is a natural remedy for increasing good cholesterol (HDL), while decreasing inflammation, body fat, blood pressure, bad cholesterol (LDL) and triglycerides. Most (not all) clean foods are found on the perimeters of the grocery store: Better yet, find out where your local farmer's market is held and buy local! Food nutrients are higher in locally farmed foods, because they can be eaten within a few days of being harvested, instead of being stored and transported long distances to the grocery store. The older the fruit or vegetable, the less micronutrients it contains.

TIP: Look at the ingredient list FIRST to determine if food is processed.

Although you may not be able to pronounce all ingredients on the list, begin the practice of observing what is in your food. Do some research to see if the food you are choosing is enhanced with vitamins and minerals, or if it's simply full of added sugar and many different preservatives that your body does not need.

A debatable contradiction is whether animal protein food sources like meat, fish, poultry, eggs and dairy (milk, butter, cream, cheese) can be considered "clean". This is secondary to how factory farms treat animals with hormones and antibiotics. These farms have elected an approach to prevent disease and maximize their growth and food output, so it is wise to know where your food is coming from. You retain the personal choice on whether you consume meat, fish, poultry, eggs and dairy, be it kosher, vegan, vegetarian, or flexitarian (flexible) diet. I recommend you choose grass fed meat, free range poultry, and organic dairy sources whenever possible.

2. Macronutrients

The three macronutrients are carbohydrates, protein, and fat; our bodies sole sources of energy or calories. The body's first priority for nutrients is to supply energy for daily functioning. Carbohydrates are sugars, starches and fiber that fuel your muscles and brain. Whole-grain breads, cereals, rice, pasta, dairy, fruits, and vegetables provide carbohydrate energy. Protein fuels muscle and tissue maintenance and recovery. Lean meat, poultry, fish, eggs, low-fat milk, yogurt, cheese, legumes, nut butter, nuts, and seeds provide protein. Fat is for energy and building healthy cells. Healthy fats come from plant based sources, such as avocados, coconuts, olives, nuts, seeds, and nut butters. Most of the population can balance energy needs as follows:

Carbohydrates = 45-65% of total daily calories
Protein = 10-35% of total daily calories
Fat = 20-35% of total daily calories

All of the macronutrients are composed of carbon (C), hydrogen (H) and oxygen (O2) which are used for energy. Protein also contains nitrogen (N) which is used to build muscle, bone, and hormones. When we are building or preserving lean body mass it is important first to get sufficient energy in our diets and enough protein to build additional muscle. Muscle building requires extra energy as well as extra protein. Your body loses muscle along with fat during weight loss. This is why it is important to boost your dietary protein while losing weight. Getting enough protein will fuel fat burning while preserving that lean muscle. [4]

3. Carbohydrates

There are three types of carbohydrates:
1. Starches-from starchy vegetables and grains.
2. Sugar-
   A. Natural sugar from whole food sources: vegetables, fruits, grains & dairy.
   B. Added sugar in processed foods.

3. Fiber-from plant foods. There is no fiber in animal sources such as milk, eggs, meat, poultry or fish.

Starches
If you put me on a deserted island and asked me to live on one food source for a long duration, I'd choose the awesome nutrition found in starchy food sources: whole grains, corn, peas, beans and root vegetables. They are most people's favorite with good reason. They are naturally packed with vitamins, minerals, complex carbohydrates and fiber! Low carb diets have given this group a bad name. Whole grains, legumes and root vegetables provide your gut with healthy microbiomes (gut bacteria). These play a role in your digestive tract metabolism and immune function.

Added Sugars (aka Free Sugars)
The Food and Drug Administration will launch a new nutrition

facts food label within the next one to five years. The new label will make it easier for consumers to make better informed food choices. According to FDA, the refreshed nutrition fact design must include the following information regarding added sugars: [5]

- "Added sugars" (in grams and as percent Daily Value) will be included on the label. Scientific data shows that it is difficult to meet nutrient needs while staying within calorie limits if you consume more than 10 percent of your total daily calories from added sugar, and this is consistent with the 2015-2020 Dietary Guidelines for Americans.
- By law, serving sizes must be based on amounts of foods and beverages that people are actually eating, not what they should be eating. How much people eat and drink has changed since the previous serving size requirements were published in 1993. For example, the reference amount used to set a serving of ice cream was previously 1/2 cup but is changing to 2/3 cup. The reference amount used to set a serving of soda is changing from 8 ounces to 12 ounces.
- Package size affects what people eat. So for packages that are between one and two servings, such as a 20 ounce soda or a 15 ounce can of soup, the calories and other nutrients will be required to be labeled as one serving because people typically consume it in one sitting.
- For certain products that are larger than a single serving but could be consumed in one sitting or more manufacturers will have to provide "dual column" labels to indicate the amount of calories and nutrients on both a "per serving" and "per package"/"per unit" basis. Examples would be a 24 ounce bottle of soda, or a pint of ice cream. With dual-column labels available, people will be able to easily understand how many calories and nutrients they are getting if they eat or drink the entire package/unit at one time.

Of all carbohydrates, added sugars are the most confusing. Added sugars include: added sugar, syrups, honey and juice, but do NOT include naturally occurring sugars found in fruit and milk. Currently, food labels only account for sugar, not added sugars.

This makes it difficult to know the difference between sugars naturally occurring in a food and those with added sugar. Until this change is made in food labeling laws (empowering informed choices for consumers) you will need to look at the ingredient list to see if these sugars are added to each food you consider purchasing. Ingredients are listed from the highest to lowest amount in order of quantity. It is strongly recommended by the 2015 World Health Organization (WHO) guidelines to reduce "added" or "free" sugar intake to less than five percent of total energy. [6] These recommendations are based on analysis of the latest scientific evidence. This evidence shows:

1. Adults who consume less sugar have lower body weight.
2. Increasing the amount of sugar in the diet is associated with a weight increase.

In addition, research shows that children with the highest intakes of sugar-sweetened drinks are more likely to be overweight or obese than children with a low intake of sugar-sweetened drinks. Sugar is over consumed by all age groups. Less than fifteen percent of people comply with the WHO's dietary advice. If you were counting grams of added sugar, here is what that might look like in one day. [2]

Children 4-6 years 19g per day ~ 4 teaspoons
Children 7-10 years 24g per day ~ 5 teaspoons
Children 11 years + and adults 30g per day ~6 teaspoon

Sugar is in most processed foods. In addition to increasing your appetite, increasing inflammation, speeding up the aging process, and decreasing your immunity, eating too many processed foods will increase your risk for illness, cancer, emotional imbalances, and weight gain-and it doesn't stop there! Food is not only affecting how we feel and our longevity, but food affects HOW we think! [7, 8, 9, 10] Our cognitive intelligence is optimized or altered with every food choice. Every single thing that we eat affects our intelligent bodies.

Below is a list of fifty most common aliases for sugar.

Note the repetitive words: sugar and syrup.

1.	Barley malt	30.	Honey
2.	Beet sugar	31.	Icing sugar
3.	Brown sugar	32.	Invert sugar
4.	Buttered syrup	33.	Lactose
5.	Cane juice crystals	34.	Maltodextrin
6.	Cane sugar	35.	Maltose
7.	Caramel	36.	Malt syrup
8.	Corn syrup	37.	Maple syrup
9.	Corn syrup solids	38.	Molasses
10.	Confectioner's sugar	39.	Muscovado sugar
11.	Carob syrup	40.	Panocha
12.	Castor sugar	41.	Raw sugar
13.	Date sugar	42.	Refiner's syrup
14.	Demerara sugar	43.	Rice syrup
15.	Dextran	44.	Sorbitol
16.	Dextrose	45.	Sorghum syrup
17.	Diastatic malt	46.	Sucrose
18.	Diastase	47.	Sugar
19.	Ethyl maltol	48.	Treacle
20.	Fructose	49.	Turbinado sugar
21.	Fruit juice	50.	Yellow sugar
22.	Fruit juice concentrate		
23.	Galactose		
24.	Glucose		
25.	Glucose solids		
26.	Golden sugar		
27.	Golden syrup		
28.	Grape sugar		
29.	High-fructose corn syrup		

Fiber

Because fiber is only found in plant based foods, being mindful of your fruit, vegetables, whole grains, nuts and seed intake can be a bowel movement game changer. Our bodies NEED 25-30 grams of fiber every single day! Not only does it help improve food satiety and insulin efficiency, it decreases arterial congestion for greater heart health. Lastly, it sweeps through your intestines like a broom giving you those daily, award winning bowel movements we can all be proud of!

4. Dirty Dozen & Clean Fifteen

The Dirty Dozen and the Clean Fifteen lists are a produce selection resource. The Clean Fifteen is not to be confused with the definition of clean eating, defined earlier in this phase. These two lists are launched annually by the Environmental Working Group. The lists are helpful in discerning which fruits and vegetables are "safer" to select if not organic, and how to best prioritize on a food budget. To get the latest information, search The Environmental Working Group at www.ewg.org or and download their "dirty dozen" app.

Just because a food is on the Dirty Dozen list doesn't mean you should never eat it. Organic is an option, but eating conventional produce is better than eating no produce! Wash your produce thoroughly, as this may help decrease your exposure to any harmful chemicals which may have been used. Note: I do not have a strict personal constituition about eating organic over conventional. However, I certainly do make a point to choose produce that's in season, regardless of whether it's organic or conventional.

The Clean Fifteen list doesn't necessarily make it top notch. Often times these make the clean list because of lower pesticide residues-so use this list as a resource, not a rule, while making informed decisions.

5. Acceptable Processed Foods (APF)

Processed food is any food that has been intentionally altered in some way prior to consumption. According to The Academy of Nutrition and Dietetics, processed food can include food that has been: cooked, canned, frozen, packaged or changed in nutritional composition (through fortifying, preserving or preparation). You can adopt the balancing notion that many foods "fit". To help with this decision-making process I have coined a technique called the APF test. APF stands for Acceptable Processed Food. First, determine if a food is processed or not. If it is processed, the nutrition facts will pass a four-itemed APF test.

This test is good for reviewing processed foods ONLY! The APF test is NOT for foods that have one hundred percent recognizable ingredients listed in the ingredient list. For example: "Brand A" peanut butter lists the following ingredients: peanuts, oil, and salt. This brand would not qualify for the APF test. On the contrary, "Brand B" peanut butter contains: peanuts, oil, salt, *sugar,* and *soy lecithin* (the last two being *food additives*). Brand A peanut butter is the better choice, because it contains less additives. Brand B is considered a processed food source. The next step would be to put Brand B to the APF test. If Brand B passes the APF test, it is considered an APF source.

Always check the ingredient list before purchase or consumption. This is one way to determine if the food contains additives and preservatives. If the food item is not processed, high five! If the food is processed, look further at the nutrition facts to see if it can be considered (what I call) an acceptable processed food (APF). This acceptability is based on the nutritional quality of the food. Clean foods are BEST, but nonetheless, nutritional processed foods can be an important and sometimes necessary part of your diet. The Nutrition Facts food label can help you determine if a processed food is an APF source, by utilizing a four-point test. To test APF sources, first check the ingredient list to be sure it is not processed.

If it is processed, but you want to purchase the food anyway, put it to this test. REMEMBER!... If you try to put non processed foods to this test, it is likely to fail. The APF test is only valid, per one serving of a processed food. If the processed food meets this four-point test, consider it acceptable, but not necessarily the BEST choice for nutrition.

You will find it beneficial to memorize the APF numbers, copy it onto a piece of paper that will live in your wallet or take a phone photo for easy access while food shopping.

Total Fat <7g	**Less than 7 grams per serving**
Saturated Fat <3g	**Less than 3 grams per serving**
*Dietary Fiber 2g or more	**2 grams or higher per serving**
Added Sugar <7g	**Less than 7 grams per serving**

Note: Dietary fiber is included for processed foods made with grains, legumes, fruits and vegetables ONLY! (i.e. breads, flavored rice and other grains, cereals, crackers, chips, canned vegetables, combination meals, such as pizza and a frozen burrito).

Do not include dietary fiber for APF analysis with protein and dairy foods such as meat, fish, poultry, cheese, butter, oil, yogurt and eggs. Naturally, animal food sources do not contain dietary fiber. Fiber is found in plant based foods. For example, processed proteins such as canned or packaged tuna, canned or packaged salmon, canned or packaged sardines, tofu, canned or packaged chicken, egg substitute, whey protein powder, yogurt, cheese, milk, and milk substitutes do not contain dietary fiber. However, total fat, saturated fat, and added sugar should come within range for processed protein and dairy foods. Total fat, saturated fat, dietary fiber, and added sugar should come within range for processed grains, legumes, fruits and vegetables.

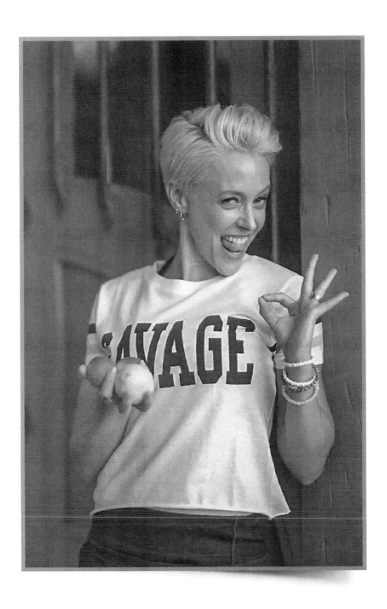

6. Sodium (Salt)

A low sodium recommendation range is between 1500-2000 milligrams of sodium per day. [11] When choosing clean most of the time, and consuming fewer processed foods, you will significantly decrease your sodium intake, as it is often found hiding there. For those that take blood pressure medications, the discontinued consumption may ultimately lead to a follow-up with your physician to verify your required dose. Talk to your doctor about the changes you are making in your diet. If you do not have hypertension and your blood pressure is at healthy levels, it is okay to add salt to food for taste. Be mindful to taste your food before adding salt. Sometimes, we are simply in the habit of adding salt, but do not actually need it for flavor.

Sodium has benefits. It assists in body maintenance of acid-base balance, regulates water in your body, stimulates muscles to contract and nerves to activate. However, when we eat too much salt our bodies hold water. A direct result of this is the increase of force against blood vessel walls. This is blood pressure. High blood pressure is a silent killer.[12] There is an increased risk of cardiovascular disease when high blood pressure goes unnoticed. If you have low blood pressure it could benefit you to increase your salt intake. Yet, be sure to increase fluid intake too, because low blood pressure correlates to being dehydrated.

Low Sodium

A food that contains less than 140 milligrams of sodium per serving is a low-sodium food. A very low-sodium food has less than 35 milligrams per serving. Foods that supply fewer than 5 milligrams per serving is considered sodium-free. Be sure to check the nutrition facts panel for the sodium quantities per serving. The food for one serving may be low in sodium, but if you eat more than the noted serving size, you will be getting more than the label defined.

Reduced Sodium

Reduced sodium is not the same as low sodium. Reduced sodium means that it has 25 percent less sodium than the amount normally found in the regular version. Don't be fooled! A reduced sodium product may still be a high sodium food! For example, soy sauce contains 879 milligrams of sodium. With 25 percent of the sodium removed, the reduced-sodium version still has about 550 milligrams. That is five times the amount of a low sodium food.

7. Alcohol

Alcohol impacts your health. In fact, its impacts are quite surprising considering many people enjoy it so frequently. To even consider limiting the intake of alcohol, most need a really good reason; the reason being as good as it is simple. Why does alcohol negatively affect your health? Allow me to air out the dirty laundry.

Alcohol is a diuretic, therefore the more you drink the more you urinate. The more you urinate, the more dehydrated you become. Excessive drinking can lead to depletion through dehydration and electrolyte imbalance. Add in the increase of the body toxin, acetaldehyde (created by the liver during alcohol metabolism) and you have a hangover. Acetaldehyde, from alcohol, is classified as a group one carcinogen. This is the same group classification as tobacco, radon, and asbestos.[13]

After a day of moderate drinking, dehydration can leave you physically and mentally fatigued. Your chances of working out the next day are reduced significantly! This is not a good recipe for fitness results!

If you do not exercise, studies show negative health benefits after the consumption of one drink (40 grams). One alcoholic drink has zero effect on the amazing hormone, testosterone. However, all effects change the more you drink.

Studies show that after three drinks testosterone decreases by twenty-three percent within 10 to 16 hours. This drop does not return to normal levels for another 36 hours. Additionally, muscle protein synthesis and leucine oxidation, which enable us to build muscle, both decrease while drinking. [14] In summary, for every drink, our energy metabolic and muscle building processes are delayed by twelve hours. All this to say, we lose one full day (24 hours) of our ability to burn energy efficiently when we consume two alcoholic beverages.

Studies show that moderate amounts of alcohol reduce the hormone, Leptin. This hormone makes us feel full. If you're trying to lose weight, overeating becomes more challenging when Leptin isn't able to do its job. [10] Alcohol affects your overall energy metabolism. Your body uses glucose and fat for energy through glycolysis and beta oxidation. However, when you drink alcohol, your metabolism shifts toward breaking down the alcohol instead. While the body is working hard to break down alcohol to a usable energy source called acetyl-CoA, everything you've eaten while drinking alcohol will be put on the back burner until the alcohol is broken down first.

One detriment to over-drinking is that alcohol decreases your quality of sleep. You may notice that you fall sleep faster at first, but are quickly disrupted because REM sleep is reduced. When we sleep, most of the recovery mechanisms are at play. Muscle synthesis, muscle recovery, and growth hormones (in my opinion, the fountain of youth), are secreted during sleep. None of this is happening while the body is intoxicated. Disrupt your sleep, disrupt your results! [11] Alcohol is one of your greatest foes to weight loss and decreasing body fat composition. However, if you do choose to drink, drink moderately. Moderate is defined as one serving of alcohol for women, per day, and two servings of alcohol for men, per day. [15]

> One serving of alcohol is:
>
> - **12 ounces of 5% beer = 1 serving (40g)**
> - **5 ounces of 12.5% wine = 1 serving (40g)**
> - **1.5 ounce of 40% liquor = 1 serving (40g)**

Women absorb and metabolize alcohol differently than men. Females generally contain less body water and higher fat percentages than men, even at a similar body weight. Therefore, women achieve higher concentrations of blood alcohol than men after drinking the same equivalent amounts of alcohol. Not to mention, women who drink more than moderately, have a higher risk of developing depression, breast cancer, liver, throat issues, and problems with wombs, ovaries and ovarian tubes. [14, 16]

Based on my professional observation, if you are willing to drink no more than three servings (recommendation for women) and four servings (recommendation for men) of alcohol *per week*, you can be successful at weight loss or weight maintenance while enjoying alcoholic beverages.

In conclusion, Phase II of *Evolve Healthy* is about being able to make informed choices. It *is not* a doctrine to be followed 100 percent of the time. Food shaming is as limiting as body shaming. Take what you need and leave the rest.

Fulfillment and happiness are not achieved by restriction, but by liberation.

References

1. Morris, A. M., & Katzman, D. K. (2003). "The impact of the media on eating disorders in children and adolescents". Pediatrics & Child Health, 8(5), 287–289.

2. Trust for America's Health. (2012, September) "F as in Fat: How Obesity Threatens America's Future", 2012. Retrieved from http://healthyamericans.org/report/100/

3. American Heart Association. (2016, August). "About Metabolic Syndrome". Retrieved from http://www.heart.org/HEARTORG/Conditions/More/MetabolicSyndrome/About-Metabolic-Syndrome_UCM_301920_Article.jsp#.Wrf-V0xFzIU/

4. Helms, E. R., Aragon, A. A., & Fitschen, P. J. (2014). "Evidence-based recommendations for natural bodybuilding contest preparation: nutrition and supplementation". Journal of the International Society of Sports Nutrition, 11, 20. http://doi.org/10.1186/1550-2783-11-20

5. FDA U.S. Food & Drug Administration. (2018, March 15). "Changes to the Nutrition Facts Label". Retrieved from https://www.fda.gov/food/guidanceregulation/guidancedocumentsregulatoryinformation/labelingnutrition/ucm385663.htm

6. World Health Organization. (2015). "Sugars intake for adults and children: Guideline". Retrieved from http://www.who.int/nutrition/publications/guidelines/sugars_intake/en/

7. Avena, N. M., Rada, P., & Hoebel, B. G. (2008). "Evidence for sugar addiction: Behavioral and neurochemical effects of intermittent, excessive sugar intake". Neuroscience and Biobehavioral Reviews, 32(1), 20–39. http://doi.org/10.1016/j.neubiorev.2007.04.019

8. Avena NM1, Bocarsly ME, Rada P, Kim A, Hoebel BG. (2008) "After daily bingeing on a sucrose solution, food deprivation induces anxiety and accumbens dopamine/acetylcholine imbalance". Physiology & Behavior., 94(3):309-15.Retrieved from https://www.ncbi.nlm.nih.gov/pubmed/18325546

9. Peet, M. (2004). "International variations in the outcome of schizophrenia and the prevalence of depression in relation to national dietary practices: an ecological analysis". Br J Psychiatry, 184:404-8. Retrieved from https://www.ncbi.nlm.nih.gov/pubmed/15123503.

10. Blancas-Velazquez A1, la Fleur SE2, Mendoza J3. (2017). "Effects of a free-choice high-fat high-sugar diet on brain PER2 and BMAL1 protein expression in mice". Retrieved from https://www.ncbi.nlm.nih.gov/pubmed/28687372

11. The American Heart Association. (2017, November 13). "Shaking the Salt Habit to Lower Blood Pressure. Retrieved from http://www.heart.org/HEARTORG/Conditions/HighBloodPressure/MakeChangesThatMatter/Shaking-the-Salt-Habit-to-Lower-High-Blood-Pressure_UCM_303241_Article.jsp#.WrgEh0xFzlU

12. The American Heart Association. (2018). "Why Blood Pressure is the Silent Killer". Retrieved from http://www.heart.org/HEARTORG/Conditions/HighBloodPressure/UnderstandSymptomsRisks/Why-High-Blood-Pressure-is-a-Silent-Killer_UCM_002053_Article.jsp#.WrgE-kxFzlU

13. American Cancer Society. (2016, November 3). "Known and probable human carcinogens". Retrieved from http://www.cancer.org/cancer/cancer-causes/general-info/known-and-probable-human-carcinogens.html

14. US. Department of Health and Human Services. (1999, December). "Are Women More Vulnerable to Alcohol's Effects?" National Institute on Alcohol Abuse and Alcoholism, No. 46. Retrieved from https://pubs.niaaa.nih.gov/publications/aa46.htm

15. National Institute of Alcohol Abuse and Alcoholism. "What Is A Standard Drink?" Retrieved from https://www.niaaa.nih.gov/alcohol-health/overview-alcohol-consumption/what-standard-drink. Accessed March 25, 2018.

16. Center for Substance Abuse Treatment. "Substance Abuse Treatment: Addressing the Specific Needs of Women". Rockville (MD): Substance Abuse and Mental Health Services Administration (US); 2009. (Treatment Improvement Protocol (TIP) Series, No. 51.) Chapter 3: Physiological Effects of Alcohol, Drugs, and Tobacco on Women. Retrieved from: https://www.ncbi.nlm.nih.gov/books/NBK83244/

Our evolution is the revolution.

-Seane Corn

Phase III: Sustenance

Sustenance is like muscle we must build to create healthy habits. It provides energy and strength needed to acquire necessary discipline. This is an intense phase, requiring careful consideration to each step. Some steps have multiple layers to review and process. You may find it relevant to spend a day on each one. After you review each step, reflect on ways to prepare to implement your plans. Document your ideas in the provided spaces. At the end of this phase, you will be prepared to begin exercising (movement). In this phase, you will be equipped to begin using the *Evolve Healthy* Food Diary located in the index of this book.

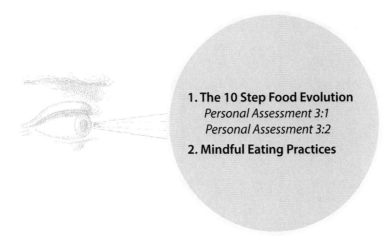

1. The 10 Step Food Evolution
Personal Assessment 3:1
Personal Assessment 3:2
2. Mindful Eating Practices

Human beings are creatures of habit; some of our habits make us happy and healthy and some do not. **People feel *successful* when engaged in behaviors that breed self respect**. Developing good habits takes discipline, courage, time, energy and sometimes, money. Setting intentions to foster postive habits will facilitate conscious action.

The word "discipline" isn't a sexy word for many people. Yet, this word has power. In Latin, *disciplina* means "teaching" and "learning". Discipline is the practice of training and obeying a system of conduct or method of practice; a code of behavior. Through correction, we learn self control to rise above, what Buddhist call, the monkey mind.

Habit formation involves stages of change. According to the Transtheoretical Model, an integrative, biopsychosocial model to conceptualize the process of intentional behavior change, the stages of change are **pre-contemplation, contemplation, determination, action, maintenance, and termination.**[1] Business Coach Tom Bartow has simplified these stages with his version called, "Three Phases of Habit Formation." [2]

1. The Honeymoon Phase: a result of something inspiring.

2. The Fight Through: a result of winning the fight to move through the struggle, making it easier to win the next one.

3. Second Nature: a result of "getting into the groove." Even though discouragement and disruptions still occur, the seduction of success begins to take over as we focus on the positive results.

Bartow notes that shifting back into phase two from phase three is normal. However, he encourages us by stating a person will make a comeback to phase three, Second Nature, after overcoming two or three more "fight throughs". Forming habits comes with consistent commitment to discipline. Discipline is what gets us past the "fight through" when we are struggling. For every endured "fight through", there is a new level of success. You may be thinking, "Why can't forming positive habits be easy?" EXCELLENCE is never easy at first, and only becomes easy when it becomes passionate and habitual. Many things worth attaining require work. Often, and more than not, attainment first endures repeatitive failure. Consider this: What is known as *failure* is simply another opprotunity to find a better way.

Below is the 10 Step Food Evolution to *Evolve Healthy.* Each step has a purpose to *identify and shift* your mental, physical, and emotional attachment to food.

The 10 Step Food Evolution:

1. Set Priorities
2. Create Meal Structure
3. Identify Motives
4. Choose Wisely
5. Be Present
6. Hydrate
7. Crave
8. Recover
9. Journal
10. Move

1. Set Priorities

Identify your priorities and you will see a direct link to how you choose to feel. The act of getting organized takes discipline. Prioritizing our load can seem time consuming, but once it's done, the task can move with greater ease. Setting priorities is a practice to set yourself up for success! Ask yourself, **"How do I want to feel after I complete my priorities?"** For example, when filling in a Proactive Plan worksheet, you are creating an intentional map to *Evolve Healthy.* Specifically, it provides a visual reminder to when you will exercise, grocery shop, meal prep, and take time for Self-care. Listing our priorities inspires us to carry out healthy decisions. Having made a decision in advance, we are more likely to follow through with our commitments! When we make ourselves a priority, we practice discerning what we really want.

The word "diet" has been abused and misused, and is long overdue for definition clarification, and meaningful reconsideration. Indeed, diet is a reference to food and drink in terms of quality, composition and impact on health. Additionally, *diet* can be a term used to reference ANYTHING we *consume* through our senses. Things like television, internet, books, social media, music, tobacco, herbs, attitudes, thoughts, people and cultures. However, the perceived and more common *interpretation* of diet, which has left a negative spin on the noun, is a selection or limitation on the amount a person may *eat* for weight reduction. Collectively, our culture does not like food limitations. Strangely, on the contrary, fad diet participation is at an all time high. The same fad diets recycle over the years with new names, and people continue to get sucked into the promises of their temporary outcomes. It seems people are addicted to the all or none principle, but this principal is rarely sustainable

NOTE: We can celebrate cultural, communal and nourishing qualities by arranging food choices and serving sizes.

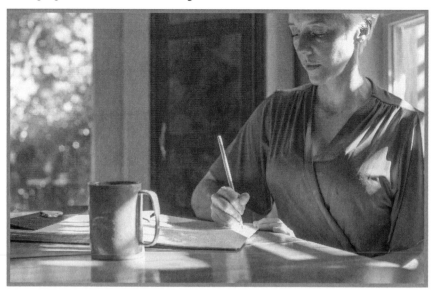

Personal Assessment 3:1

Do your current priorities align with what you really want?

1. What do you CURRENTLY consider your top 5 priorities?

1. _____

2. _____

3. _____

4. _____

5. _____

2. What do you WANT (not should) your top 5 priorities to be?

1. _____

2. _____

3. _____

4. _____

5. _____

3. Do they align? If not, what will it take to align them?

2. Create Meal Structure

Meal Times

It takes the human body about two to three hours to digest a moderate-sized meal. There are two meal interval options to consider for meal structuring:

1. Fed State

2. Post-absorptive State

Let's look at the first meal interval option. **A fed state promotes eating every two to three hours.** To remain here, you are always in the process of digesting food. The benefits to this? Your hunger levels never peak. Eating more frequently, however, does not necessarily increase your metabolism. What this *can* do, is keep you focused on eating the right foods *before* the state of hunger hits, and boundaries of self-discipline are crossed with poor food choices. It is a good strategy to consider eating every two to three hours if the following needs describe you:

1. You tend to eat generous portions when you get hungry.

2. You tend to feel powerless over food choices due to your hunger, thereby eating unhealthy, quick and convenient foods.

3. You like to graze throughout the day on very small portions.

4. You are an athlete who must eat more often to train efficiently.

A post absorptive state promotes eating every four to five hours. In this state, your body will utilize stored energy reserves *after* it has digested your former meal. Hormone levels adjust to shift from "fat storage mode" into "fat-burning mode".

Post-absorptive state may reduce free radical damage and inflammation while increasing the production of anti-aging hormones and the promotion of tissue repair. This state may also protect you from developing diabetes as the body stabilizes baseline blood sugar levels between meals.

In my professional opinion, it serves to balance these two states. **The median interval of eating every 3-4 hours works for many of my clients.** Eating a moderate meal every 3-4 hours is practical. However, one size never fits all. Please note that eating every 2-3 hours, 3-4 hours, or 4-5 hours is completely safe and effective if YOU find it sustainable! Your metabolic rate can remain healthy through either state. Recognize there is NO suggested meal timing of "5 plus" to "6 plus" hours between meals. Normalized hunger patterns occur about every 3-5 hours. However, life does happen and your body can adjust. The exact hourly interval will depend on individual body composition, daily activity, genetics and the type of fuel used to feed it.

Personal Assessment 3:2

What meal intervals do you think would work best for you? Choose a clock time that reflects your *ideal* meal timing schedule.

Meal 1 _____ am/pm

Meal 2 _____ am/pm

Meal 3 _____ am/pm

Meal 4 _____ am/pm

Meal 5 _____ am/pm

Meal 6 _____ am/pm

Food Grouping

The following recommendation for food grouping is taken from my eBook, *The Mindful Clean Plate.* [3]

Choose different food groups at each meal.

A modest meal consisting of two (minimum) to five (maximum) *different* food groups will provide a variety of macronutrients at each meal. This is to say, that each food group contains no more than one serving each, per meal. Although, having two servings may be beneficial if you need more food. A food group is a category in which different foods are placed according to their type of nourishment (see Food Groups list in index).

There is an emphasis on the word, "different." Repeating the same food group at one meal (serving both berries and a banana) would NOT be wrong, but indicative that the same food group has been repeated. To repeat a food group at a meal is not a problem, but dividing the fruits into one-half servings, thereby creating one, would better vary nutrients. Ultimately, this means you feed yourself more micronutrients with less total caloric intake. The balancing intake of essential vitamins and minerals becomes easier. Additionally, choosing a variety will also balance macronutrients (carbohydrates, proteins, and fats).

For example:

1 banana + a handful of almonds =2 different food groups ("FG").
1 C oatmeal + 1 C berries +1 handful of walnuts= 3 FG.
3 oz. chicken +1 C spinach +1 C brown rice+1 tsp sesame oil= 4 FG
(If I added 1 C of peaches to the last meal, I would then have 5 different food groups.)

For the average, healthy adult trying to lose weight, and gain lean muscle mass, it is recommended that no more than 30 grams of quality lean protein is consumed *per meal*, three to four times a day. (90-120 grams daily total)

Animal protein sources come from meat, fish, poultry, eggs low fat diary, and whey protein powders. Plant based proteins come from legumes (beans), lentils, mycoprotein, seeds, nuts, tofu, tempeh, and pea protein powders. Choosing lean protein at most of your meals, including breakfast, will promote greater muscle protein synthesis. Protein intake doesn't necessarily mean protein availability. Therefore, if you are vegan, you will need to eat about ten percent more plant based protein sources than the animal protein recommendation. This is because the protein in plants have less bioavailability. (amount of protein your system is able to absorb).

Another benefit to varying food groups is a natural balancing of the endocrine hormone, insulin. Insulin is responsible for regulating blood glucose levels and involved in the regulation of how your body uses and stores fat. Glucose, known as blood sugar, is the result of broken-down carbohydrates. Carbohydrates are found in ALL foods, excluding eggs, meat, fish and poultry (those that once had eyeballs). Think of insulin like Uber®. Uber® is a car service that provides "reliable rides in minutes". Insulin, like Uber®, swiftly transports broken-down carbohydrates where they need to go. Insulin drops off glucose at the following locations:

"House" #1 - blood
"House" #2 - muscle
"House" #3 - liver
"House" #4 - fat stores (adipose tissue)

Some cells in the body can take glucose from the blood without insulin, but most require that it arrives via transport. When we habitually exercise, eat moderate-sized meals and are mindful of meal timing, we are teaching our cells to uptake glucose without insulin. This doesn't mean insulin is obsolete, only that our body does not require as much for homeostasis. That is nothing short of awesome! This means that when we eat, food gets to go wherever it needs to go without Uber®...I mean insulin! It's almost like magic.

The "magic" I am referring to is actually called GLUT4 protein. GLUT4 protein is the insulin-regulated glucose transporter found primarily in adipose tissue and striated muscle (both skeletal and cardiac). See why it's easier to just call it…magic? Anyway, when you exercise regularly, GLUT4 protein increases, thereby being more readily prepared to take blood sugar where it needs to go. Studies show that acute exercise enhances muscle GLUT4 protein translocation. Exercise creates a rapid increase in magic… I mean, muscle GLUT4 protein! My point is, exercise proves again to be magical! Research concludes that exercise can play an important, if not essential role, in the treatment and prevention of insulin insensitivity. [14] Insulin insensitivity can be likened to be calling for Uber which then shows up late, or not at all. With more GLUT4 in our bodies we transport glucose energy all by itself. Here is the best part- with more "magic" (Glut4 protein) and less "Uber®" (insulin) congesting our "highways" (blood supply), the fewer House #4 (fat) stops by glucose energy!

Below are my suggested food grouping blueprints based on the average energy needs of an adult. First, discern what you are trying to accomplish: weight loss, lifestyle maintenance, or increased performance. If you desire to lose weight, choose the *weight loss* blueprint. If you desire to maintain a healthy weight, choose the *lifestyle* blueprint. If you are a recreational or competitive athlete (physically training for performance, up to or exceeding 9 hours per week), choose the *performance* blueprint. All blueprints suggested will need to include an additional post workout recovery meal. This will be discussed in step 8, *Recover*. Please note, that this is a suggestion for those recovering from diet culture, but aren't sure how to transition to intuitive eating. As you practice these boundaries, you may find it easier to blend or expand your blueprint as you experience changes in your mindset and body. For best results, document your mealtimes and food choices in their correct food group using the *Evolve Healthy* Food Diary found in the index of this book.

- **Weight loss- Choose 2 -3 different food groups every 3- 4 hours.**
- **Lifestyle - Choose 3-4 different food groups every 3-4 hours.**
- **Performance - Choose 5- 6 different food groups every 3-4 hours.**

*All blueprints: For best results, at every meal, choose lean protein (animal or plant based) or low fat dairy, as one of your food groups.

Other notable considerations:

- Protein from meat, fish, poultry, legumes, and dairy are slower to empty from the stomach, thereby increasing satiety.

- Fats from nuts, seeds, avocados, olives, and oils are slower to empty from the stomach, thereby increasing satiety.

- Non-starchy vegetables: All veggies that are not "starchy vegetables" fall within a flexible or "free" food group (see Food Groups list in index). The flexibility offered by this group invites you to count these vegetables as one of your different food groups, or not. Permission slip: Over consume vegetables as desired. Always feel liberated to eat more veggies!

- Stop eating 2-3 hours before you lay down to sleep. While many have fallen prey to the myth that eating before bed makes you fat, this is not scientifically true! This suggestion is made because your body requires adequate time for full digestion, allowing you to gain the most from your sleeping hours. Quality sleep (7-9 hours per day) will provide restoration and adequate generation of hormones (such as growth hormone most active during slumber) that balance and aid in anti-aging.

- If you experience an intolerable hunger within those last two hours before bed, first try drinking a tall glass of water. If that doesn't satisfy you, choose vegetables, lean proteins, or whole grains

3. Identify Motives

For those who experience emotional or physical challenges regarding eating, food, and distorted self-image, a new philosophy is shaped with simple shifts in thought patterns. What we think about food is based on our life experiences. *Recognizing* what thoughts provoke emotions, thereby causing a "food reaction", is a game changer. By observing the ways you cope with your emotions, you may begin to re-think your food choices. Recognizing this difference is vital to choosing foods without the limiting emotional influences of shame, blame and guilt. We must be willing to understand why we eat what we eat, when we eat it. A powerful question to ask yourself is, **"What are my motives for eating this?"** Sometimes, you may find your body needs fuel, while other times, it's just for sport. That's right, for **SPORT**. If only the common thrill of eating was a sport... wait... it is! Okay, well... extreme competitive eating is not healthy either, so I digress. The point is, when we shift our thinking to "food is fuel", it still houses the ability to invoke feelings of nostalgia and joy. This is a healthy motivation to eat.

As discussed in Personal Assessment 1:3, identifying a craving as emotional or physiological can be challenging. A question to ask yourself is, **"Is my hunger a sign that I need to be distracted or that I need to refuel?"**

Here are three mindful eating questions to ask yourself, to identify your cravings as a "need for comfort" or a "need for nourishment".

1. What am I hungry for?

2. What am I feeling right now?

3. Where do I feel this emotion inside my body?

Question 1: What am I hungry for?

Try this next exercise on your own, with your *Evolve Healthy* partner, or small group. One of the group members may read aloud the questions, as the others answer them internally, or aloud if appropriate. Afterwards, document your observations.

- Before eating, sit down in a chair with awareness to posture.
- Sit tall, if you can.
- Close your eyes and take two deep breaths.
- Ask yourself the question, **"What am I hungry for?"**
- Give yourself one full minute here.
- Observe your thoughts and feelings.
- Does your focus go toward your body?
- How does it feel within the gut region?
- Does an emotion arise?

If your body is communicating it needs nourishment, then it is best to feed it. If it is the *body* that is hungry, *not* the mind, then it is time to eat. If you are unsure, that is okay. Not everyone has this ability to tune-in right away and could have a lack of awareness. This could also come from years of ignoring signals. Others lack the ability due to an imbalance in hormones. *Regardless*, continue asking the questions. Live in the questions. As you gain greater awareness of the mind, awareness of the body will follow.

A balanced body will give you physical symptoms of hunger. Physical signs of body hunger can be experienced through mind-body awareness. **Because the body follows the mind, being aware of your body is essentially being in TUNE with your mind.** With practice, you can become aware of HOW your body is doing on the inside. Once you become aware, you begin to move toward syncing the mind with your physiological body. The body raises two red flags when needing fuel:

1. The stomach will feel like an empty pit. It may or may not grumble. To observe this emptiness, try this:

- ✔ Go into your gut with your mind's eye (visualize your stomach).
- ✔ Close your eyes.
- ✔ Breathe in gently, and concentrate on the oxygen entering the body through your nose. Bring your focus into your stomach.
- ✔ What do you sense there?

2. Dizziness, extreme irritability, sweating, lethargic, inability to concentrate, nausea, and headache are classic symptoms that a hormone imbalance has occurred secondary to not eating. These imbalances occur when we have not listened to the first sign of hunger. If we resist eating when the body signals, the body will continue to communicate to the brain that it is time to eat.

Question 2: What am I feeling right now?
Try this...

- ✔ Before eating, sit down in a chair with awareness to posture.
- ✔ Sit tall, if you can.
- ✔ Close your eyes and take in two deep breathes.
- ✔ Next, ask yourself the question, "What am I feeling right now?"
- ✔ Give yourself one full minute here.
- ✔ Observe your thoughts.
- ✔ Does an emotion come to mind?
- ✔ Name it.
- ✔ **Say it out loud!**

With practiced awareness, you will begin revealing the emotions that impact your choices. If the feeling is neutral or positive, you will more likely exercise self-discipline with food choices and portion control. An individual's connection to emotions and food choices are as unique as you are. Being aware of your current emotional status will help you identify any trends around eating behaviors. Once you recognize a trend, you are better equipped to transcend the behavior by choosing differently. The simple act of becoming AWARE of the "wanting" provides a GAP for change, acceptance, or removal that you may choose to evolve! (C.A.R.E.)

Question 3: Where do I feel this emotion inside my body?

If you recognized an emotion from the previous question, you are ready for the follow up.

> ✔ Maintaining that same seated posture, close your eyes, and ask yourself, "Where do I feel this emotion inside my body?"
> ✔ Give yourself one full minute here.
> ✔ Observe your thoughts as you scan the body.
> ✔ Place your hand on the specific body part or region where you are experiencing the emotion(s).
> ✔ Breathe deeply into this area of your body.
> ✔ Then, affirm to yourself, "It's okay to let 'this' go."

If more emotions arise, allow them to come. Some may be uncomfortable, even unbearable, but stuffing or ignoring them altogether is never successful. They only make or keep you sick. You are sacred and worthy of this attention. Feeling these may be the very key to your breakthrough! Sometimes, these emotions only need surface for a moment. Look them dead in the eye and say, "I see you." Like short-staying visitors, invite the experience in, and they will soon be on their way. Let them come. Let them go. Each time you practice, this will get easier, and you will arise stronger with greater tolerance to the turmoil that inevitably visits us all, from time to time.!

Do what you can to keep conversations neutral and light while you eat. While these will inevitably be experienced, negative emotions disrupt the diamagnetic flow of digestion in the body, causing indigestion and other forms of unease within the gut. If possible, steer clear of negative emotions while eating (frustration, anger, anxiety, and confusion to name a few). If you find you are eating with unpleasant emotions, then STOP! Push the food aside and be with your emotions instead. Return to your food when you feel ready.

*Refer to the chakra chart in Phase I for introspection.

Choose Wisely

At this point, you are in full swing of food prepping and weekly grocery store shopping as instructed in Phase II. If not, make it your priority to begin no later than NOW! Food freedom breeds choice! How fantastic is it that you get to choose what to eat?! Your choices are negotiable, and you call the shots! You can choose healthy, clean, whole, cooked, raw, fast, junk or processed foods whenever you want to! It's true! This is a privilege and a right, thank goodness!

BE PROACTIVE-NOT REACTIVE! Regardless of whether the food is healthy or not, proactive choices offer confidence and opportunity. Reactive choices are more likely to offer those false, limiting emotions: shame, guilt and blame. Ask yourself, **"How do I want to feel after I eat?"** Ideally, you will choose optimally and fuel your body for health. The reality is that sometimes you will not. I encourage you with all of my heart to enjoy your choice, even if it's unhealthy from time to time. Making this mental effort is a part of your evolution to heal the source fracture story around food and body image.

Be Present

The act of eating can become an art form! To be mindful is to be present in the moment. Remaining present while eating promotes greater nutrient absorption and overall nourishment. When we simply eat, while we eat, we do so more slowly. The art of eating, in presence, will take you approximately 10-30 minutes. Think of what you do during a meal. Consider this…stop multitasking and be with your food.

STOP eating and watching TV.

STOP eating and checking social media notifications.

STOP eating and reading.

STOP eating while tending to emails.

STOP eating and working.

STOP eating while talking on the phone.

STOP eating and driving.

STOP eating and planning.

STOP eating and…

Try sitting (or standing) while you eat mindfully, savoring every glorious moment. I would like to re-introduce you to two of the most simple, mindful eating practices: table manners and your five senses. "Minding your manners" can help define the meaning of your meal. Eating is a physical need, but meals are a social ritual. Many of us learned these as a young child, but either lack of practice, or sheer rebellion, have kept us far removed from their contribution to mindful eating. Consider table manners and observing your five senses a vehicle into presence while eating.

Witnessing all five human senses while eating is quite the trip. Often, I find myself shoveling down my food and I miss the bliss of observation. When I tune in and focus on my senses, my food is ingested and digested more kindly. I cannot help but be in the NOW when observing my senses.

Try this next exercise on your own, with your *Evolve Healthy* partner, or small group. One of the group members may read the instructions aloud. Afterwards, document your observations.

Before you begin this mindful eating exercise, prepare yourself a treat. It could be as simple as one berry, or a piece of chocolate. Set an intention to romance every bite. With child-like wonder, observe your five senses as if they were brand new to you.

1. Observe- Literally look as if studying or seeing food for the first time.

2. Smell - Take one deep breath; enjoy its natural aroma before taking your first bite.

3. Touch- Before you taste, and if appropriate, touch your food.

4. Taste - Chew and swallow slowly; feel the movement from your throat into your stomach.

5. Listen - Hear the biting sensations and enjoy them in your head as you chew.

Other mindful eating practices that bring presence to your meal:

- Take a sip of water between each bite.
- Place your eating utensil down between each bite.
- Close your eyes when you are tasting the flavor.
- Chew and swallow slowly before attempting to get the next bite ready.
- Move slowly as you transition: from a bite of food, to a sip of your beverage, to the use of your napkin, etc.
- Take small bites
- Observe your stomach expanding. This expansion is a physical communication to you to note when it is time to STOP eating. If you resist this signal, you may eat more that your body needs.

Even if you are dining alone, take the opportunity to practice these mindful eating exercises, also known as manners.

Before you eat:

- Wash your hands.
- If dining with others, kindly wait until everyone has arrived, sitting and served before you begin. ESPECIALLY offer this courtesy towards your cook, should they be joining you. This most simple expression of awareness extends your offering of appreciation and respect towards their time, talent and efforts without ever speaking a word.
- Offer a blessing of gratitude, for both your food, and the hands that prepared it (this can be silent or aloud, individually or collectively).
- Place your napkin on your lap.
- Take a moment to really see your food.
- Consciously inhale and take in the aroma of your food.

During your meal:

- Sit or stand with good posture if possible. If seated at a traditional dining table, place both feet on the ground, with your chair drawn in towards the table. Your spine should be long and lifted. If standing, position yourself to face your food, in lieu of leaning on the counter.
- Bring the food to your mouth, not your mouth to the food.
- Lean towards your plate without rounding into it. One reason "no elbows" are to the table, is that it avoids the tendency to perch upon them. Resting forearms encourages posture, and keeps you from getting too close to your plate.

- Select small bites that will allow you to comfortably chew with minimal effort.
- Chew slowly and thoroughly. Smaller bites digest more easily, so take your time and don't scarf your food.
- Chew with your mouth closed. If your bite requires your mouth be open, you are most likely taking too big of a bite. Please consider those across from you as well. No one wants to see, or hear, everything you are enjoying.
- Refrain from speaking while food is in your mouth. Whatever you need to say can wait. Again, consider those you are speaking to. They want to hear what you have to say, and it is MUCH clearer when your mouth is free of food. Should it be you find yourself at a business luncheon where time is limited and you really need to be able to eat (and speak), then consider your order AND the portion sizes you collect upon your fork.
- Consider speaking only when spoken to. This eliminates excess ingestion of air, which may cause gas. A meal shared will provide ample time for both parties to speak and eat.
- Cover your mouth if you must speak, burp or sneeze. This is where that handy-dandy lap napkin serves you well.
- Wipe your mouth with a napkin.

After your meal:

- Fold your napkin and place it to the left of your plate.
- Take a moment before standing to savor what you just experienced.
- Stack dishes neatly.
- Clean your space.

Hydrate

Did you know you need to consume the water equivalent (in ounces) of half your bodyweight per day? For example, if your weight is 130 lbs. your daily needs are 65 ounces. of water. Do the math and write your needs below. Next, consider getting a handy dandy, re-usable 24+ounce bottle. Commit to carrying this with you everywhere you go. Think of it as the new friend who is readily offering a source of vitality that pushes you towards meeting your needs. You will urinate more, but think of it as a gentle, purifying cleanse. This "release" will cleanse from the inside out, while increasing your metabolic rate. Water is responsible for several metabolic processes including, digestion, waste management, and temperature regulation. Adequate water makes everything in your body operate better—**EVERYTHING!**

Daily Hydration Needs

A SEDENTARY, non-exercising body, needs its body weight, (in pounds) divided by two (in ounces) per day.

Pounds of body weight _____ / 2 = _____ounces of water that I need each day for a sedentary lifestyle.

Exercising adults need to add an *additional* one to two liters to meet their daily need. [4] Are you surprised? Remember, you are ORGANIC! Think of how a plant looks when deprived of water. Like humans, a plant's water needs vary by size.

About twenty percent of your daily fluids come from food. Most fluids you drink count towards hydration, including milk, juice, carbonated water, diet or regular soft drinks, kombucha, smoothies, coffee and tea. (Note: regular consumption of high concentrated juices and soft drinks are not reccommended). Instead, choose pure, plain water, over flavored beverages most of the time. I often hear people remark that unflavored water is boring. If you feel like you are 'addicted' to flavored beverages, begin with setting a goal to limit them. Instead, try adding flavorful, hydrating foods that are helpful, such as fruit slices, cucumbers or lemon juice. NOTE: Sports drinks may be necessary for endurance athletes that exercise intensely for 90+ minutes, per session. Consult with your sports dietitian for further recommendations.

NOTE:
Excess caffeine and alcohol robs your organs of water and dehydrate the body. [5]

Caffeine

If you drink more than one cup (8 ounces) of any caffeinated beverage per day, be sure to drink more water throught the day.

Research shows that hydration status is unaffected by consuming up to 400 milligrams of caffeine per day.

How many ounces of caffeinated beverage do you drink each day? _____

How many ounces of water do you need based on your body weight? _____

Add the above two numbers together

My daily fluid needs are _____

Alcohol

If you drink more than one serving (see page 57) of alcohol per day, add an additional 8 ounces of water for every one serving of alcohol.

How many servings of alcohol do I drink each day? _____

How many additional ounces of water do I require? _____

Add this number to your daily fluid needs based on your body weight, and any extra fluids needed secondary to extra caffeine consumption.

My daily fluid needs are _____

Track Your Hydration

The *Evolve Healthy* Food Diary provides a hydration tracking system. Droplets are provided at every meal entry. Each droplet represents eight ounces. If you drink eight ounces at a meal, check off, or color in one droplet; for 16 ounces, check off two droplets, and so on. If you drink in between meals, great! Track these too! Tracking will create accountability for adequate consumption. Soon it will soon become a habit to drink more throughout the day.

Crave

Crave, a verb defined by Merriam-Webster, means "an intense, urgent or abnormal desire or longing for (something)." [6] Most commonly craved foods are high in empty calories. Empty calories means it has no substantial nourishment to the body. **Cravings are most often driven by habit.** Overindulgence effects ninety-seven percent of Americans. Research shows that while desire may *feel* irresistible, we are more strongly influenced by context, habit and conditioning [7]. This is stellar news! We can retrain our appetites thereby reducing cravings! When it seems like there is nothing to do but give into your cravings, THINK AGAIN! By training your cravings you are no longer a slave to your appetite.

How to Retrain Your Cravings

Own your cravings, then choose wisely. Next, take conscious action and choose what foods you desire. Throughout the week, pay attention to what types of foods you are craving. When the day of your Mod-Meal arrives, ask yourself BEFORE you go out to eat, attend an occasion/event, or go to the grocery store, the following questions:

1. **What foods am I craving right now?**
2. **What foods do I truly want to experience?**

Do NOT negotiate your Mod-Meal choices with others. It is critical that this "training process" is completed without the influence of others. Trust yourself as you make your own empowered choices. If you "cheat" by adding an additional Mod-Meal, "fall off the wagon," or feel as though you have in any way "slipped, missed the mark, or failed", I urge you to contemplate (without judgment) why this *needed* to happen. **Drop the guilt.** Your awareness is required to learn from an experience. Take time to reflect and consider how you can better prepare for the next compelling desire. It is going to be okay! This is how we learn. Get back to choosing healthy options as soon as you can.

Until we adopt the motto on a cellular level, "**choices lead and feelings follow**", we need self-compassion to catch us when we fall. Your feelings are valuable. They are a natural fact of life and can serve as magical pointers to personal triggers. It is our feelings that compel us to consume or purge. Although, feelings are a part of us, they do not need to lead the way when a choice is made to fill an emotional lack caused from negative thinking. **Likewise, guilt is stifling and shame has NO productive insights for change.**

My body has knowledge and it reminds me that the temporary joy that arrives from large portions is rarely worth it. Eating for *sport* cannot keep us fulfilled for very long. However, please be gentle with yourself as you slip, stumble, fall, leap, duck, dodge and triumph. They are evolutionary steps in your progress. It all matters and is worthwhile. Keep going! You have come this far. You are blazing your trail to well-being.

Recover

Whether you are a weekend fitness warrior or a seasoned athlete, eat a recovery meal after a moderate to intense workout. During exercise exertion, your body uses stored muscle energy called glycogen. A prime energy source during moderate to intense activity, glycogen is stored glucose from carbohydrates eaten prior to workouts. It is the body's fuel that is ready for action! **Topping off glycogen stores is vital for your next physical activity or performance.** You want to show up with your storage tanks full! If you do not, you tucker out more quickly, muscles burn more readily, and your mental focus becomes skewed. We need to fill our glycogen tanks because, unlike stored fat, glycogen is energy on demand. Furthermore, think of it as an insurance policy for your next workout. The next time you are intensely lifting weights, climbing a rock wall, paddling a kayak, or running those hills, you will be glad you invested in your glycogen storage!

Recovery nutrition affects how your muscles and connective tissues heal. [8] While glucose from carbohydrates are necessary to replenish glycogen stores, protein is necessary for muscle recovery. By eating a post workout meal, we greatly reduce the risk of chronic fatigue in future workouts. Moreover, we reduce the metabolic burning of muscle tissue, instead of body fat! To be strong and energetic follow these post-workout, recovery-nutrition guidelines:

1. Eat carbohydrates and protein directly after your workout; the sooner the better. If you can eat within 15-45 minutes of completion, do it! OPTIMAL RECOVERY comes from eating within that window of time! If that is not possible, do it as soon as you can. Glycogen will be replenished, and your tired muscles will begin to rebuild and repair with the necessary protein and amino acids.

2. Your body is more likely to store food as glycogen instead of fat, directly after intense activity. Therefore, after a workout would be a great time to have a Mod-Meal. Furthermore, after an intense athletic session, added sugars may aid in quicker recovery.

3. Choose recovery meals that contain carbohydrates, proteins, and help rehydrate. Examples:

- Smoothie made with low-fat milk (or plant based non-dairy source) and fruit
- Protein powder with water and fruit
- Low-fat chocolate milk
- Turkey on a whole-grain wrap with veggies and yogurt
- Yogurt, berries and water
- Fruit, nuts and low-fat cottage cheese
- Boiled eggs, avocado, brown rice and water
- Celery, peanut butter and fruit
- Carrots, hummus and string cheese
- Coconut water and pistachios
- Cucumber, tuna fish and plain low-fat yogurt

Journal

Journaling creates accountability, behavior modification and thus trains the mind. [9] When we choose to make a record, we choose mindfulness. Documenting your food intake and emotional observations will serve you well in your progression to *evolve healthy*! Emotional journaling helped me get through some sticking points while recovering from my eating disorder. Even now, when I notice myself reverting to the "fight thru" phase of creating habits, I journal. Every time I write, my awareness grows. It helps me see what I need to see and shift perspectives, if desired. Many of my clients have had life-changing discoveries journaling their emotions.

Food Journaling: The *Evolve Healthy* food diary's sole purpose is to empower food grouping and timing, while bringing awareness to your choices and emotions. This food diary is for you to NOTICE your choices. Note: If at anytime the food diary becomes irritating, too cumbersome, or makes you feel disempowered or deprived, please STOP using it. Instead, consider emotional journaling.

Write directly onto the pages, of your *Evolve Healthy* Food Diary found in the index of this book. If you are a planner, go ahead and plan your day inside your journal entries, but WRITE IN PENCIL! Provide space for life to happen. Be flexible and kind to yourself as prior made decisions may change. I recommend you print five to seven days worth of blueprints for the week. Staple them together, fold them into a booklet and keep it in a place that is easily accessible, like your pocket, purse, lunch bag or backpack.

Note: A 24-hour food recall is not the best way to document compared to journaling as-you-go. Eating and recording food while in the present moment, will provide reflection over reaction to thoughts. Many observations can be found hidden in the moment, while others will be noticed at the end of the day, week, month, or year. Documenting allows you to look for trends that point to common denominators. Common denominators can look like a feeling, a need, a want, or a strategy used to meet a need or a want. The reflective nature of journaling provides a safe place to learn about your patterns.

The index of this book includes fillable *Evolve Healthy* Food Diary blueprints to get you started. **Additional copies of this diary can be downloaded at www.MindfulBodyRevolution.com** Each page includes two journal entries; two plates per page. Each plate represents one meal. Additionally, each entry includes two questions to ask yourself prior to eating! **"What am I feeling right now?"**, and **"Where do I feel this in my body?"** The more awareness you have, the more nourishing your food can be. If you choose unhealthy foods, write it down; observe why this might have occurred, then love it too. If you are not sure which group to place your food, it is better to guess than to not participate. However, if you know for certain that a food does not belong in a food group, for example: chocolate cake written into the dairy group, refrain from writing it there. Instead, use the blank lines or the blank space around the blueprint, to document choices that are not whole foods.

Review the hand written food diary examples on the following pages.

How to use the
The **Evolve Healthy Food Diary**

Be sure to Write date at the first meal of each new day

Document Clock time at each meal

Circle each time you document a new meal

Circle each time you document a new meal

Date: __/__/__   Time: _____ AM / PM meal time
Day: M T W Th Fri Sat Sun
Meal: 1 2 3 4 5 6 7

Date: __/__/__   Time: _____ AM / PM
Day: M T W Th Fri Sat Sun
Meal: 1 2 3 4 5 6 7

WATER

Check 1 droplet for every 8oz of water consumed at each meal + between meals

WATER

Choose your correct food grouping range. i.e. 2-3 food groups every meal.

(1) DAIRY 4oz Cottage cheese

FAT

Free Food group

DAIRY

FAT

PROTEIN | VEGETABLE

NOT FREE FOOD group
☐ STARCHY VEGETABLE

PROTEIN | VEGETABLE

☐ STARCHY VEGETABLE

(2) 7 WHOLE GRAIN crackers | (3) 1c. FRUIT pineapple

Check to acknowledge when documenting

WHOLE GRAIN | FRUIT

Space to document "junk food"

Close your eyes for a few seconds when asking yourself this question.

What am I feeling right now?
Love / Mad / Glad / Happy / Sad / Scared / Confused / Other

Where do I feel this inside my body?
_____
_____
_____
_____

What am I feeling right now?
Love / Mad / Glad / Happy / Sad / Scared / Confused / Other

Where do I feel this inside my body?
_____
_____
_____
_____

→ Space to document workout / movement

→ Space to document observations + celebrations

The **Evolve Healthy Food Diary**

Date: **3/1/XX**   Time: **6:25** (AM)/ PM
Day: (M) T W Th Fri Sat Sun
Meal: (1) 2 3 4 5 6 7

WATER *16 8 H2O + 1 mug of coffee*

DAIRY — *2 T. 90 cottage cheese*

FAT

PROTEIN — *1 egg*

VEGETABLE

☐ STARCHY VEGETABLE

WHOLE GRAIN — *1/2 c oatmeal*

FRUIT

What am I feeling right now?   *Content*
Love / Mad / Glad / Happy / Sad / Scared / Confused / (Other)

Where do I feel this inside my body?
upper abdomen.
Mind is calm

Date: __/__/__   Time: **10:30** (AM)/ PM
Day: (M) T W Th Fri Sat Sun
Meal: 1 (2) 3 4 5 6 7

WATER *16 8 H2O*

DAIRY — *1 c. Greek yogurt*

FAT — *1 oz almonds*

PROTEIN

VEGETABLE

☐ STARCHY VEGETABLE

WHOLE GRAIN

FRUIT — *banana*

What am I feeling right now?
Love / (Mad) / (Glad) / Happy / Sad / Scared / Confused / Other

Where do I feel this inside my body?
All over!
I was hungry!
I couldn't eat until 10:30 but was
hungry at 9:30 am.

The **Evolve Healthy Food Diary**

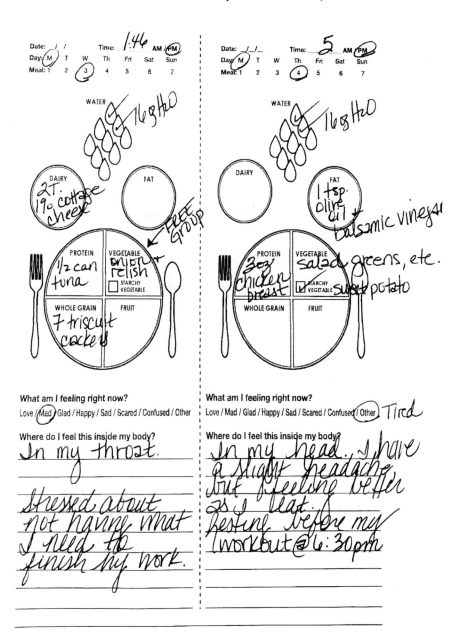

Date: / /   Time: 1:46 AM (PM)
Day: (M) T W Th Fri Sat Sun
Meal: 1 2 (3) 4 5 6 7

WATER — 16g H2O

DAIRY
2 T.
1% cottage cheese

FAT

FREE Group

PROTEIN
1/2 can tuna

VEGETABLE
onion relish
☐ STARCHY VEGETABLE

WHOLE GRAIN
7 triscuit crackers

FRUIT

What am I feeling right now?
Love / (Mad) / Glad / Happy / Sad / Scared / Confused / Other

Where do I feel this inside my body?
In my throat.

Stressed about not having what I need to finish my work.

Date: / /   Time: 5 AM (PM)
Day: (M) T W Th Fri Sat Sun
Meal: 1 2 3 (4) 5 6 7

WATER — 16g H2O

DAIRY

FAT
1 tsp. olive oil + balsamic vinegar

PROTEIN
3 oz chicken breast

VEGETABLE
salad greens, etc.
☑ STARCHY VEGETABLE sweet potato

WHOLE GRAIN

FRUIT

What am I feeling right now?
Love / Mad / Glad / Happy / Sad / Scared / Confused / (Other) Tired

Where do I feel this inside my body?
In my head. I have a slight headache but feeling better as I eat. Resting before my workout @ 6:30pm

The **Evolve Healthy Food Diary**

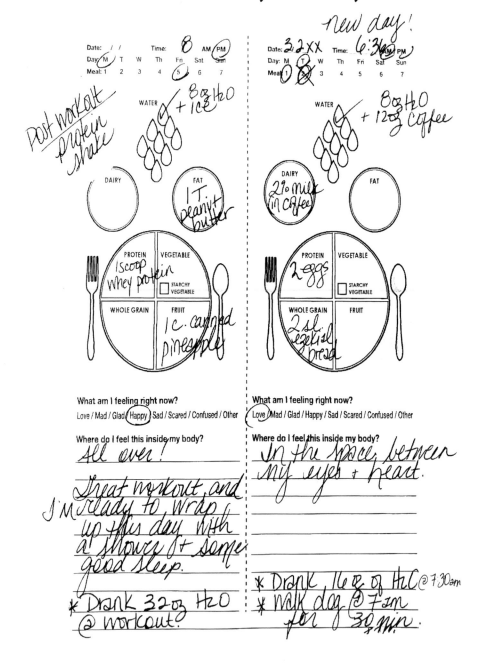

Date: / /   Time: 8   AM (PM)
Day: (M) T W Th Fri Sat (Sun)
Meal: 1 2 3 4 (5) 6 7

new day!

Date: 3.2.XX   Time: 6:36 (AM) PM
Day: M (T) W Th Fri Sat Sun
Meal: (1) (2) 3 4 5 6 7

Post workout protein shake

WATER   + 8oz H₂O + ice

WATER   8oz H₂O + 12oz Coffee

DAIRY

FAT   1 T. peanut butter

DAIRY   2 oz milk in coffee

FAT

PROTEIN   1 scoop whey protein

VEGETABLE

☐ STARCHY VEGETABLE

WHOLE GRAIN

FRUIT   1 c. canned pineapple

PROTEIN   2 eggs

VEGETABLE

☐ STARCHY VEGETABLE

WHOLE GRAIN   2 sl. ezekiel bread

FRUIT

What am I feeling right now?
Love / Mad / Glad / (Happy) / Sad / Scared / Confused / Other

What am I feeling right now?
(Love) / Mad / Glad / Happy / Sad / Scared / Confused / Other

Where do I feel this inside my body?
All over!

Great workout, and I'm ready to wrap up this day with a shower + some good sleep.

* Drank 32oz H₂O @ workout.

Where do I feel this inside my body?
In the space between my eyes + heart.

* Drank 16 oz of H₂O @ 7:30am
* walk dog @ 7am for 30 min.

The **Evolve Healthy Food Diary**

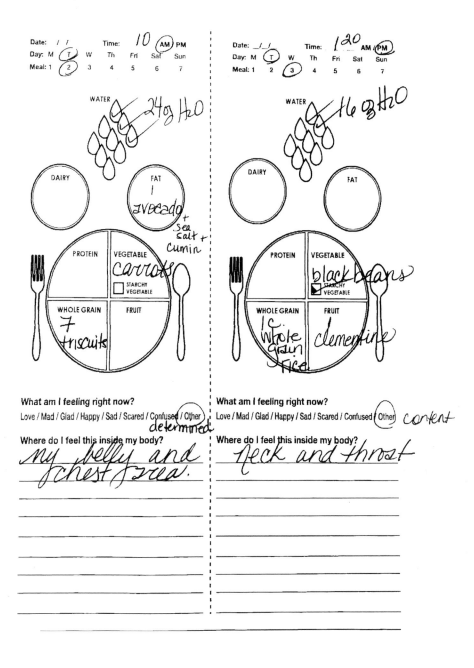

Date: / /   Time: 10 AM PM
Day: M (T) W Th Fri Sat Sun
Meal: 1 (2) 3 4 5 6 7

WATER — 24 g H2O

DAIRY

FAT
1
avocado + sea salt + cumin

PROTEIN   VEGETABLE
carrots
☐ STARCHY VEGETABLE

WHOLE GRAIN   FRUIT
7 triscuits

What am I feeling right now?
Love / Mad / Glad / Happy / Sad / Scared / Confused / (Other)
determined

Where do I feel this inside my body?
my belly and chest area.

Date: _/ /   Time: 120 AM (PM)
Day: M (T) W Th Fri Sat Sun
Meal: 1 2 (3) 4 5 6 7

WATER — 16 oz H2O

DAIRY

FAT

PROTEIN   VEGETABLE
black beans
☑ STARCHY VEGETABLE

WHOLE GRAIN   FRUIT
1 C. whole grain rice   clementine

What am I feeling right now?
Love / Mad / Glad / Happy / Sad / Scared / Confused / (Other) content

Where do I feel this inside my body?
neck and throat

The **Evolve Healthy Food Diary**

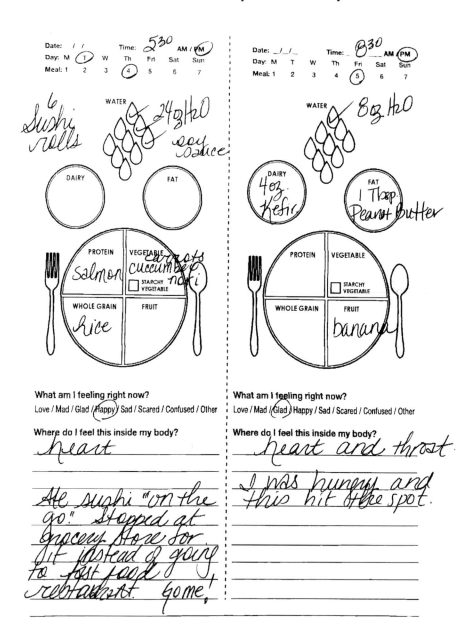

Date: / / Time: 530 AM / PM
Day: M (T) W Th Fri Sat Sun
Meal: 1 2 3 (4) 5 6 7

6 Sushi rolls

WATER 24g H2O
soy sauce

DAIRY

FAT

PROTEIN — Salmon
VEGETABLE — carrots cuccumber nori
STARCHY VEGETABLE

WHOLE GRAIN — rice
FRUIT

What am I feeling right now?
Love / Mad / Glad / (Happy) / Sad / Scared / Confused / Other

Where do I feel this inside my body?
heart

Ate sushi "on the go." Stopped at grocery store for it instead of going to fast food restaurant. Go me!

Date: _/_/_ Time: 830 AM / (PM)
Day: M T W Th Fri Sat Sun
Meal: 1 2 3 4 (5) 6 7

WATER 8g H2O

DAIRY — 4 oz. Kefir

FAT — 1 Tbsp. Peanut Butter

PROTEIN
VEGETABLE
STARCHY VEGETABLE

WHOLE GRAIN
FRUIT — banana

What am I feeling right now?
Love / Mad / (Glad) / Happy / Sad / Scared / Confused / Other

Where do I feel this inside my body?
heart and throat.

I was hungry and this hit the spot.

The **Evolve Healthy Food Diary**

new day.

Date: 3/31/XX   Time: 6:18 (AM) PM
Day: M   T   (W)   Th   Fri   Sat   Sun
Meal: (1)   2   3   4   5   6   7

WATER — 16 oz H₂O + coffee

DAIRY
1/2 + 1/2 creamer in coffee

FAT
2 T. Peanut Butter

PROTEIN | VEGETABLE
STARCHY VEGETABLE
WHOLE GRAIN — 2 slices ezekial bread | FRUIT

What am I feeling right now?
Love / Mad / Glad / Happy / Sad / Scared / (Confused) / Other

Where do I feel this inside my body?
In my head.
Had bad dreams
last night that
have me feeling
confused.

Date: __/__/__   Time: 10 (AM) PM
Day: M   T   (W)   Th   Fri   Sat   Sun
Meal: 1   (2)   3   4   5   6   7

WATER — 16 oz H₂O

DAIRY
1 oz cottage cheese   ←→ mix together

FAT
1 T. Peanut Butter

PROTEIN | VEGETABLE
STARCHY VEGETABLE
WHOLE GRAIN | FRUIT — apple

What am I feeling right now?
Love / Mad / Glad / (Happy) / Sad / Scared / Confused / Other

Where do I feel this inside my body?
my whole body.
I love this food
combo! ♥ PB!

The **Evolve Healthy Food Diary**

Post workout meal.

Date: _/_/_   **Time:** 2   AM /(PM)
Day: M   T (W) Th   Fri   Sat   Sun
Meal: 1   2 (3) 4   5   6   7

Salad and Protein Shake (in shaker cup)

WATER — *16 oz H2O*

DAIRY

FAT — *1 tsp. oil,*

PROTEIN — *whey powder — 1 scoop*

VEGETABLE — *Salad greens + balsamic vinegar 1 c.*

☑ STARCHY VEGETABLE — *garbanzo beans*

WHOLE GRAIN

FRUIT — *1/4 c. raisins*

What am I feeling right now?
(Love)/ Mad / Glad / Happy / Sad / Scared / Confused / Other

Where do I feel this inside my body?
All over! I feel nourished + emotionally content.

worked out at lunch break (1pm)
* Drank 24 oz H2O at workout.

Date: _/_/_   **Time:** 6   AM /(PM)
Day: M   T (W) Th   Fri   Sat   Sun
Meal: 1   2   3 (4) 5   6   7

WATER — *24 oz H2O*

DAIRY

FAT

PROTEIN — *Salmon 5 oz. (grilled)*

VEGETABLE — *asparagus*

☐ STARCHY VEGETABLE

WHOLE GRAIN — *black rice 1 c.*

FRUIT — *1 c. fresh cherries*

What am I feeling right now?
Love / Mad / Glad /(Happy)/ Sad / Scared / Confused / Other

Where do I feel this inside my body?
Deep into my abdomen.

The **Evolve Healthy Food Diary**

new day

Date: __/__/__   Time: **8 25** AM (PM)
Day: M   T   W   Th   (Fri)   Sat   Sun
Meal: 1   2   3   4   (5)   6   7

WATER *14 oz H2O*

DAIRY

FAT *fridos*

combo fad

PROTEIN *1 boiled egg*

VEGETABLE

☑ STARCHY VEGETABLE *fridos*

WHOLE GRAIN

FRUIT

+ small bowl of Fridos

What am I feeling right now? *lonely*
Love / Mad / Glad / Happy / Sad / Scared / Confused /(Other)

Where do I feel this inside my body?

*In my head...
I got hungry
because I was
feeling lonely
was I even
hungry? I don't
know right now, but
my choices were
not to bad —
progress!*

Date: **3 4, XX**   Time: _____ AM / PM
Day: M   T   W   (Th)   Fri   Sat   Sun
Meal: (1)   2   3   4   5   6   7

WATER *8g H2O + 1 mug of coffee*

DAIRY *19o milk*

FAT

PROTEIN

VEGETABLE

☐ STARCHY VEGETABLE

WHOLE GRAIN *1.5 c. Cheerios*

FRUIT *1c. raspberries*

What am I feeling right now? *Content*
Love / Mad / Glad / Happy / Sad / Scared / Confused /(Other)

Where do I feel this inside my body?

my heart

The **Evolve Healthy Food Diary**

Date: __/__/__   Time: 9:45 (AM) PM
Day: M T W (Th) Fri Sat Sun
Meal: 1 (2) 3 4 5 6 7

WATER
24g H2O

DAIRY
8 oz. greek yogurt

FAT
1 oz. walnuts

PROTEIN | VEGETABLE
STARCHY VEGETABLE
WHOLE GRAIN | FRUIT

What am I feeling right now?   stressed
Love / Mad / Glad / Happy / Sad / Scared / Confused / (Other)

Where do I feel this inside my body?
My throat.

Date: __/__/__   Time: 1:__ AM (PM)
Day: M T W (Th) Fri Sat Sun
Meal: 1 2 (3) 4 5 6 7

WATER
(Chicken salad)   16g H2O

DAIRY

FAT
1 oz. walnuts

4 oz. PROTEIN canned chicken | VEGETABLE chopped broccoli
STARCHY VEGETABLE
WHOLE GRAIN | FRUIT grapes

What am I feeling right now?   stressed
Love / Mad / Glad / Happy / Sad / Scared / Confused / (Other)

Where do I feel this inside my body?
My neck + shoulders

*was able to walk after lunch. 20 min. Drank add'l 16 g H2O.

The **Evolve Healthy Food Diary**

new day!

Date: _/_/_   **Time:** _5_ AM /(PM)
Day: M   T   W   (Th)   Fri   Sat   Sun
Meal: 1   2   3   (4)   5   6   7

Planned
MOD
MEAL

WATER   ✓ _16 oz H2O_
_+_
16 oz Soda

DAIRY

FAT

PROTEIN   _burger_

VEGETABLE   _lett. tom onion_

STARCHY VEGETABLE

WHOLE GRAIN   _Bun_

FRUIT

+fries, soda, Ketchup

What am I feeling right now?
Love / Mad / Glad /(Happy)/ Sad / Scared / Confused / Other

Where do I feel this inside my body?
my head.
I have been
looking forward
to this meal & I
feel a little icky
but I'm aware
I'll recover fast
b/c I don't eat red
meat often.

Date: _/_/_   **Time:** _6:40_ (AM)/ PM
Day: M   T   W   Th   (Fri)   Sat   Sun
Meal: (1)   2   3   4   5   6   7

WATER   ✓ _8 oz H2O +_
coffee

DAIRY   _2 T._
1 oz cottage
cheese

FAT

PROTEIN   _2 eggs_

VEGETABLE

STARCHY VEGETABLE

WHOLE GRAIN   _1 c._
oatmeal

FRUIT

What am I feeling right now?
Love / Mad / Glad / Happy / Sad / Scared / Confused /(Other)   _Rushed woke up late!_

Where do I feel this inside my body?
my chest +
stomach!

The **Evolve Healthy Food Diary**

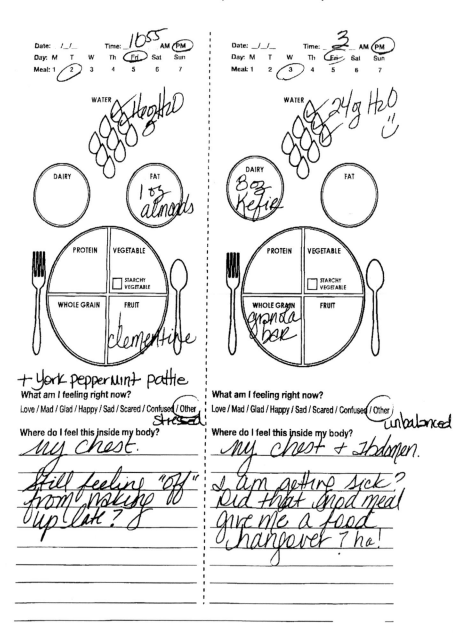

Date: /_/_ Time: 10⁵⁵ AM (PM)
Day: M T W Th (Fri) Sat Sun
Meal: 1 (2) 3 4 5 6 7

WATER *Hot H₂O*

DAIRY

FAT *1 oz almonds*

PROTEIN | VEGETABLE
STARCHY VEGETABLE
WHOLE GRAIN | FRUIT *clementine*

+ York peppermint pattie

What am I feeling right now?
Love / Mad / Glad / Happy / Sad / Scared / Confused / (Other)
stressed

Where do I feel this inside my body?
my chest.
still feeling "off"
from waking
up late?

Date: /_/_ Time: 3 AM (PM)
Day: M T W Th (Fri) Sat Sun
Meal: 1 2 (3) 4 5 6 7

WATER *24g H₂O*

DAIRY *8 oz Kefir*

FAT

PROTEIN | VEGETABLE
STARCHY VEGETABLE
WHOLE GRAIN *granola bar* | FRUIT

What am I feeling right now?
Love / Mad / Glad / Happy / Sad / Scared / Confused / (Other) *unbalanced*

Where do I feel this inside my body?
my chest + abdomen.
I am getting sick?
Did that food meal
give me a food
hangover? ha!

The **Evolve Healthy Food Diary**

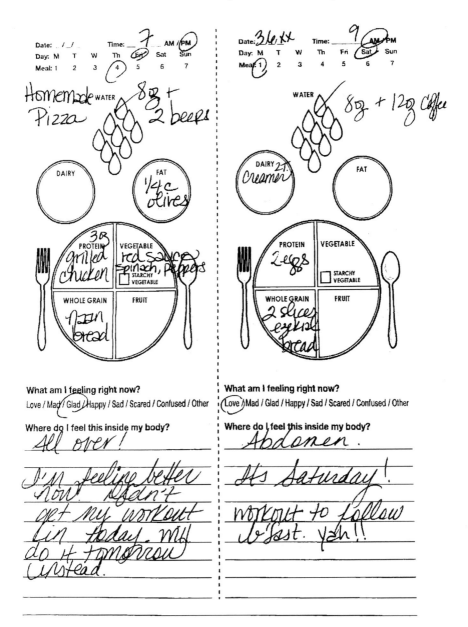

Date: _/_/_ Time: _7_ AM /PM
Day: M T W Th (Fri) Sat Sun
Meal: 1 2 3 (4) 5 6 7

Homemade WATER 8ჳ +
Pizza 2 beers

DAIRY

FAT
1/4 c
olives

3ჳ
PROTEIN
grilled
chicken

VEGETABLE
red sauce
spinach, peppers
STARCHY
VEGETABLE

WHOLE GRAIN
thin
bread

FRUIT

What am I feeling right now?
Love / Mad / Glad / Happy / Sad / Scared / Confused / Other

Where do I feel this inside my body?
All over!

I'm feeling better
now. didn't
get my workout
in today. will
do it tomorrow
instead.

Date: 3/6/xx Time: _9_ AM /PM
Day: M T W Th Fri (Sat) Sun
Meal: (1) 2 3 4 5 6 7

WATER 8ჳ + 12ჳ Coffee

DAIRY 2T.
Creamer

FAT

PROTEIN
2 eggs

VEGETABLE
STARCHY
VEGETABLE

WHOLE GRAIN
2 slices
ezkiel
bread

FRUIT

What am I feeling right now?
Love / Mad / Glad / Happy / Sad / Scared / Confused / Other

Where do I feel this inside my body?
Abdomen.

Its Saturday!
workout to follow
b'fast. yah!!

Move

Conscious movement will strengthen your mind, body and spirit! It's not what you do, it's how you do it. Move with intention. Find something that sparks internal joy while doing it. Carve out time for movement most days. "Move it or lose it" is truth. If you are going to move your body to increase your heart rate, choose something that you enjoy, sparks joy and can be accomplished daily.

If you are currently uncertain or without preference, I will take this moment to encourage you with great passion. As a Certified Strength and Conditioning Specialist and Yoga teacher, I highly recommend that at least 120 minutes of your 150-320 total minutes, be dedicated to resistance training (i.e. weight training) and Yoga. The remaining time can be more cardiovascular focused, such as walking, running, dancing, etc.

Resistance training has beneficial effects on power, strength, flexibility, speed, health, speed, body composition, and fitness.[10] Resistance training can include anything that provides tension. I love lifting weights and practicing Yoga. I am not sure which one I love more, and thank goodness I don't have to choose, but I'd like to invite you to try Yoga if you have not already. You do not have to be physically flexible to benefit. Albeit, flexibility, is a side effect.

Coming to your mat to breathe with others is witnessing an entire room of souls breathing together as ONE. It's so beautiful. Yet, do not mistaken, Yoga is not for the weak hearted. Sweat? Yes. Also, there are tears, moans, breakdowns, and breakthroughs. Yoga is for those that are willing to trek the wild, juicy, and even grotesque parts of yourself. For myself, and many, it's about inner work. At the right time, and especially if you're open to it, your suppressed bullshit stories will bubble up. Right there on your mat, in a room filled with moving bodies who understand what's happening. Right there in that uncomfortable, stinging, intense asana (pose) that you would rather get the hell out of. You'd rather cut and run than bear witness to its sensation—it's knowledge. It's message.

Yoga is for those that don't mind getting deep into the messy middle. Not to fix it, but to meet it with love and understanding. Your body remembers everything! Every grace, every fear, every experience. The glorious mess of who you are is stored in your body. Every childhood emotion is there. That little child who didn't know what to do with her big feelings. It's still in there. They are safe there in your body for the keeping—ready to be released when you're able to acknowledge that you've disassociated from that part of yourself. You didn't know any better. Your body remembers every trauma, secret, resentment, insecurity, lover, bond, and act of deceit. You can not escape yourself—but don't we sure try. Yoga is a way to take you deeper into your pain, conscious or unconscious pain, so that the story can be told, and tension can be released. And, it is there that you will find YOUR truths and even YOUR purpose. It's hard and it sucks, but it's LIBERATION! Yoga invites you to acknowledge, own, and meet your pain with understanding. So that we might move toward empathy and forgiveness.

Ⓢ SWEET SPOT:

1. Go take a yoga class.
2. Clean out your kitchen cupboards! Discard or donate any tempting foods that you feel powerless over at this time. Grab some empty boxes and garbage bags and *do it to it!* Use your intuition. Inspired by Marie Kondo's book, *The Life Changing Magic of Tidying Up*, hold each food item in your hand and ask yourself, **"Does this food need to live here with me?"**

I believe that creating an empowering space allows for our truest self to emerge, without the clutter that can weighs us down. We do not have to store food (or any other thing) that we may use later. Buy only what you need each week. If it's Mod-Meal foods, buy those on the day of your Mod-Meal and not before. This will keep unnecessary temptation out of your home. You may find this process evolves into other areas of your life: non-edible, personal belongings, clothes, papers, and keepsakes. Let go. It is said, "Fruit that clings to the tree, rots."

References

1. Prochaska JO1, Velicer WF. (1997) "The transtheoretical model of health behavior change". Am J Health Promot. Sep-Oct;12(1):38-48. Retrieved from https://www.ncbi.nlm.nih.gov/pubmed/10170434

2. *Forbes.* Selk, Jason. Habit Formation: "The 21 day Myth". Retrieved from https://www.forbes.com/sites/jasonselk/2013/04/15/habit-formation-the-21-day-myth/#5e824d71debc Assessed March 25, 2018.

3. Fryer, J. Danielle, RDN, CSCS. (2017). "The Mindful Clean Plate". Retrieved from http://www.MindfulBodyRevolution.com/books

4. Popkin, B. M., D'Anci, K. E., & Rosenberg, I. H. (2010). "Water, Hydration and Health". Nutrition Reviews, 68(8), 439–458. http://doi.org/10.1111/j.1753-4887.2010.00304.x

5. Robert Swift, M.D., Ph.D.; and Dena Davidson, Ph.D. "Alcohol Hangover Mechanisms and Mediators". Retrieved from https://pubs.niaaa.nih.gov/publications/arh22-1/54-60.pdf. Accessed March 25, 2018.

6. Merriam-Webster. Crave. (2018, March 27) Retrieved from http://www.merriamwebster.com/dictionary/crave.

7. McGowan, Kat. (2013, August 9). "Why we Crave". *Psychology Today.* Retrieved from https://www.psychologytoday.com/us/articles/200308/why-we-crave

8. Demling, R. H. (2009). "Nutrition, Anabolism, and the Wound Healing Process: An Overview". *Eplasty*, 9, e9.

9. *Harvard Health Publishing.* (2012, March 2). "Why behavior change is hard - and why you should keep trying". Retrieved from https://www.health.harvard.edu/mind-and-mood/why-behavior-change-is-hard-and-why-you-should-keep-trying. Accessed January 19, 2017.

10. *Human Kinetics.* "The Importance of health, fitness, and wellness: Foundations of Professional Personal Training with DVD by canfitpro". Retrieved from http://www.humankinetics.com/excerpts/excerpts/the-importance-of-health-fitness-and-wellness. Accessed March 21, 2018

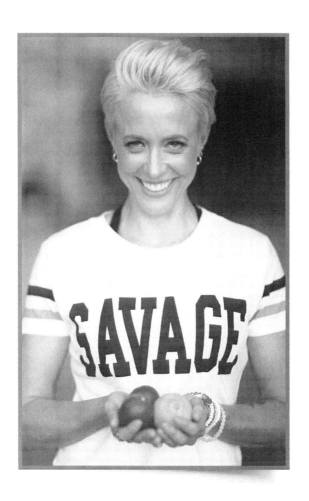

Your task is not to seek love, but merely to seek and find all the barriers within yourself that you have built against it.

-Rumi

Phase IV: Introspection

The purpose of this phase is to guide you back to into the arms of *yourself*! To practice introspection is to visit with your mental and emotional processes. This includes your thoughts, emotions, will and choices. To examine yourself is like giving yourself permission to dive into deep waters, even when you feel like only dipping in your toes.

This phase may feel tough at times. Many of you will want to put the book down and process what will be asked of you. Some of you will want to throw the book across the room and never pick it back up again! If you feel overwhelmed, please seek further support and accountability from a professional life coach, licensed counselor, or psychotherapist. Yes, it may hurt to consider many of the questions here, but I assure you, it's your truths that lead to your healing. Anything short of this phase will leave you susceptible to returning to old patterns. Choose now; dive in and experience the depth that resides within your heart. **We must feel it to heal it.**

While discerning what is true for you, personal assessments will help guide you. This self inquiry opens a way to expand with creativity and liberation.

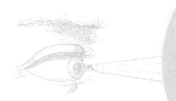

1. **Breaking Unhealthy Habits**
2. **Perception**
3. **Finding Inner Peace**
4. **Being Intentional**
5. **Setting Goals**
6. **Managing Expectations**
7. **Mindful Rituals**

Part 1. Breaking Unhealthy Habits

We all have habits, whether healthy, neutral or unhealthy. To break any habit, we must recognize how our thoughts and feelings are relating to one another. Eckhart Tolle reminds us, "Awareness is the greatest agent for change."

Meditation is a mindfulness practice that aids in sensing habit loops. Practioning meditation is like coming home to yourself; being with your thoughts, emotions and behaviors *as they are*, <u>not</u> as you *want* them to be. You do not have to sit cross-legged on the floor and burn incense, but it is okay if you do! You may sit comfortably anywhere or take a walk. I endearingly call that a *meditation in motion*.

According to psychiatrist and neuroscientist, Judson Brewer, MD, PhD, we have a natural, reward-based learning process called positive and negative reinforcement. In his book, *The Craving Mind,* he explains the **Trigger--Behavior--Reward-- Repeat** behavioral process.[1] He explains what is happening when we are trying to focus, but our attention drifts off to a completely different thought. Sudden urges arise to indulge one of our habits, like checking the phone notifications, biting nails or eating when we're not hungry. Our challenge in making great decisions, like choosing healthy foods and exercising daily, can be understood with neuroscience. The primal brain (which runs most of your life) is more concerned with playing it safe within a "comfort zone". The primal brain is reflexive, emotional and non-rational.

A trigger begins as a thought and an emotion is spawned from that thought. Simultaneously, it is experienced as a *body sensation*. **A behavior is a learned reaction to the trigger.** Brewer notes that triggers are usually from the past; a fear-based memory. A reward, however, validates the behavior (making you feel good) sometimes instantly. [1]

Example 1:

Trigger: You have a disagreement with a coworker- you feel angry.

Behavior: You go home from work and drink an entire bottle of wine.

Reward: Now relaxed from the alcohol, you feel good.

Example 2:

Trigger: You're not sticking to your healthy meal plan - you feel guilty and ashamed.

Behavior: You sabotage and pull into the fast food drive-through.

Reward: You feel satisfied from increased brain dopamine and serotonin levels.

The primal brain, tries to control our behaviors, but is not always successful. Intellectually, we know we should not eat a whole pint of ice cream. The hiccup is that this primal part of the brain can go offline when it gets stressed out! [1] When this happens, we return to old habits. This is why we need to teach ourselves how to connect and dissatisfy ourselves from poor behaviors, and instead, learn how to satisfy ourselves with healthy ones. [1]

Before getting taken for a ride by a craving, we can practice neutralizing our mental triggers. This is *best done* when we get stressed. In that moment, see if you can observe your thoughts while sensing what is happening in your body. Allow all your feelings, but mind your actions, and pay attention to what is happening in the moment. Brewer encourages us to remember that when we get *curious* about our stressful thoughts and feelings, we create an opportunity to **step out of our habit loop.** To notice our trigger is key! A pause deactivates the stressful sensory information we are experiencing. Pausing allows for a positive mental correction that is then integrated within the Cerebral Cortex of the brain. The Cerebral Cortex is conscious thought, memory, language, creativity, decision making, movement, conscious sensation and vision. [2]

If you detect a trigger, but then decide to act out on a habitual behavior, at least do it with your fullest attention! Let's say you are a binge eater who longs to quit. You notice the urge to binge, and despite your "desire to stop", decide to binge anyway. Mindfulness encourages us to be fully engaged in the experience. Observe all five senses while you binge. Perhaps, you will notice your bites are bigger and you chew faster than normal. Your stomach swells, and the food begins to smell and taste less appealing. This mindfulness technique *may* create dissatisfaction of the behavior, and **lack of satisfaction naturally leads to letting it go.**

Here's how you do it: First, start noticing your mental triggers and where you feel them in your body. Is there tightness, tension, restlessness, boredom, anger, tears, or a need for blood curdling screams into pillows? Remember, there is no wrong feeling! Stop wishing it away while stuffing it down to numb it, drugging it to dumb it, or blaming it on other people. The next time you have the urge to act out in a way that is destructive to your (and others) physical, mental or emotional well-being, try tuning into your senses and asking yourself, **"Is this thoughtful, helpful, intelligent, neutral and kind?"**

T-H-I-N-K

T thoughtful
H helpful
I intelligent
N neutral
K kind

Think of something that triggers a behavior; something that is real for you in your current life situation. Close your eyes and concentrate on it for ten seconds, or for as long as you can before another thought hijacks that one. Next, ask yourself the below questions. It is best to do this work with your partner, small group, or professional therapist.

Trigger:

What is the trigger?

What emotion is present now?

Where do you feel it in your body?

Behavior:

What do you normally do when you feel this way?

Do you take action to inhibit or enhance this behavior?

Describe it.

Reward: (feels good)

What part of that behavior gives you the gratification you are needing?

Curiosity: (Curiosity can later replace behavior and is naturally rewarding)

Why do you think that triggers you in the first place?

Is this an old fear-based wound?

Are you willing to see this differently?

Good work! I know that wasn't easy. How do you feel now?

A conscious breath is a vehicle back into the present moment.
Take a deep breath now. Breathe all the way down into your feet.

You may not yet know HOW to see it differently. The ability to see it differently takes time, and time takes time. Living in the questions of **"What am I feeling?"** and **"Where does it live inside me?"** can gently initiate the process, and move you towards, "HOW." Come back to this page tomorrow and revisit the same questions with a different trigger. Document your responses again.

Trigger:

What is the trigger?

What emotion is present now?

Where do you feel it in your body?

Behavior:

What do you normally do when you feel this way?

Do you take action to inhibit or enhance this behavior?

Describe it.

Reward: (feels good)

What part of that behavior gives you the gratification you are needing?

Curiosity: (Curiosity can later replace behavior and is naturally rewarding)

Why do you think that triggers you in the first place?

Is this an old fear based wound?

Are you willing to see this differently?

Part 2. Perception

The practice of recognizing emotions inside your body will help you connect with your physical body triggers. Triggers point to what needs your loving attention. If you want personal growth, getting curious about your "mind-made stories," is non-negotiable. This is not to say that your stories are not absolute truth, but unresolved past experiences spawn emotions that impact you and others around you. It can hurt when you detach from the painful stories. This unraveling and stripping of perception may leave you feeling naked and even angry at first. It is said that "the truth will set you free, but first it will piss you off." Although it may hurt to give up your familiar coping mechanisms, but the pain is worsened when living with mental narratives that keep you knotted up inside. A binding can loosens when you begin asking, **"What am I believing to be true that doesn't serve me?"**

I recently found myself sitting alone with an amazing view of a lake. I was all wrapped up in my mind about if I had made the right decision to move back home to Alabama after being gone for seventeen years. My throat tightened, tears were born, and my teeth clenched. I noticed body sensations of fear and sadness. I was creating a story in my mind, which boiled down to a fear of missing out. This "FOMO" (fear of missing out) was me missing sunny Arizona. I was staring directly at a beautiful Alabama lake, but I was not really seeing the lake at all. When I noticed this occurring, I took a breath and I *saw* the lake. I realized, I am right here now-*this* is what it *is*, RIGHT NOW. I giggled a cosmic giggle. I noticed my trigger, got curious about where it came from, then felt the joy of letting it go. (Cosmic giggles are a sure thing.). Glory, glory! We get to choose, over and over (possibly a few million times a day) to live in the stories or choose what is... right *NOW... NOW... NOW!*

I don't know about you, but I tend to want answers and solutions ASAP! I feel the need for a plan of action, a solution, and if possible, a *Disney* ending. As a culture, we feel the need to produce, produce, produce…and don't miss a thing going on "over there." We have a tough time living in the moment, because we are programmed to *want it all.* Your personal effort to heal the painful stories of your past, offers *everything.* It offers freedom.

I came to a point in my life where I vowed to myself that when I am triggered, I refuse to avoid it, stuff it down with food, or use other forms of numbing vices. It's not always peaceful looking, either. Ask anyone that knows me. But, I think, at least more times than not, I am present to what is happening *to me,* in the moment it is happening *FOR ME!*

 ## Sweet Spot

Narrative mode writing is a literary device that explores your inner voice expressed through a dialogue or a monologue. This writing exercise is a way to unload your stream of conscious; your present thoughts and feelings. Sit down with the next two blank pages and a pen. Allow your pen to write every single thought as it comes through your mind. Even if there is a random and seemingly pointless thought that arises, write it!

Example:

"I am being pulled in three directions. I was told to write my feelings and I really need to go to bed. This is bullshit. I'm still angry about his decision to show up like he did. I'm so tired and I want him to understand. I need to prep the coffee"…

See, it's random! This unpacking on paper can reveal what is REALLY renting mental space in your head.

Tip: Just write! Don't think about what to write, just write what is on your mind NOW! Try to write faster than you can think and let it all come out on paper.

There is no wrong way to write this, nor is there a wrong emotion, idea or conflict. By allowing our thoughts and feelings to flow onto paper, we are able to find connections between our thoughts and actions. Permission to unload here. There may be leaps between thoughts, misspellings, and no correct punctuation in your writing. Be uninhibited and stand in your authenticity as you write. Experience the release as you purge it out on paper.

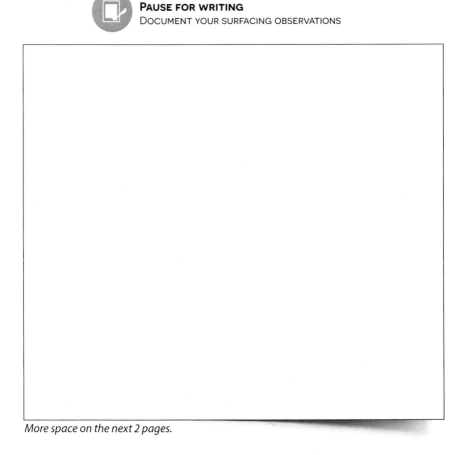

PAUSE FOR WRITING
DOCUMENT YOUR SURFACING OBSERVATIONS

More space on the next 2 pages.

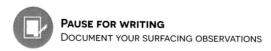

PAUSE FOR WRITING
DOCUMENT YOUR SURFACING OBSERVATIONS

Part 3. Finding Inner Peace

We can never fill the Divine hole in us; not with food, people, places or things. The God of our own understanding has already filled that space. It's taken! Yet, we try to cram other things in there that leave us feeling empty after the initial (and TEMPORARY) fill up. We will never obtain it *our way*. Each time you feel the trigger in your body and identify the mind's story that created the body sensation, ask God *to show you more*. Ask to be seen as *you are* in the moment you feel triggered. Our perception of ourselves is often blurry and self-righteous. Divine guidance can reveal our best self when we ask to see. *Ask,* then listen to this inner voice. This voice is oftentimes quiet, yet sharp; do not mistaken its edge, for it is healing. It miffs us many times, and saddens us others. It can frightens and confuse our ego. But, if inner peace is truly your goal and you want to heal, a*sk the Divine Teacher.*

What would happen if we gave up our mind-made stories? What would happen if we gave up the need to be right? To let go of conditioned thoughts, we must first learn to catch the thoughts as they arise. **Self-inquiry is the opposite of depression.** This is the way to inner peace, to surrender, to freedom and to love. The word "surrender" used to scare me. I would think, "NO WAY, I will fight till the bitter end for what I believe to be RIGHT!" What I learned was that surrender does not mean submission. Surrender means that you stop fighting with reality and stop trying to do God's part. Surrender often looks like a focused action on your part. Surrender is a *clear* choice made for yourself rather than going along with something (or someone) in order to dodge conflict or discomfort.

Everything can change around you. Your friends, spouse, job, account balance, home and health can all change in a blink. However, inner peace is a status that can be experienced anywhere, at any time. One of my favorite teachers, Byron Katie, said, "Peace is always on the inside. **Where have you been looking?"**

Give yourself permission to feel inner peace. Whisper, "My goal is inner peace," and observe how you can choose to surrender to *what is*. There may be some resistance at first, but stay with the whisper, "My goal is inner peace."

When I am triggered I ask:

- "God, show me."
- "God, use me"
- "God, help me see this differently."
- "God, is that true?"
- "God, thank you for showing me my wound(s)."
- "God, shift me now."
- "God, I ask you now for a miracle."

I get triggered every day! I'm human! In fact, most of us are triggered if we spend time around any one person, groups of people or watch television. (Especially the news.) The truth is, that triggers will never stop because *the work is never done!* My triggers have seasons where they are ripe for the pushing, while others seem less and less painful. I know they've lost their power over me when I can talk about them without tears, anger or frustration. My food and body image triggers remain, silently in my head, despite writing a book about them! What's become different over time is my reaction to them. I don't have to go off the deep end in attempts to ignore it, punish it, or revert to my old patterns of instant gratification. I am healing every time I simply TRY to see it differently, and you are too.

A decision to practice self inquiry takes humility. Humility means we recognize that we are dependent on others and on God. As we recognize our humility, we can learn to accept our shortcomings. Next, we can release it to Divine Grace. Humility expands our inner strength. When we have humility, it is because we have chosen to surrender. When we surrender, we experience inner peace. When we experience inner peace, we no longer feel the urgency to restlessly push for an outcome. There is grace, restoration, and true power in this type of surrender; here we experience satisfaction. With satisfaction, we no longer feel the need to stuff our empty spaces with things, people, food, behaviors, projects, etc. We no longer feel led to overeat, over exercise, or overachieve. When we are satisfied we don't feel the need to perform to earn our place in this world. This doesn't mean we do not set goals and work towards them. Instead, we reach for our goals from a place of passion. That passion that says, **"I will go for it, and I will be okay no matter what the outcome."** On the contrary, an attachment to an outcome says, "I will go for it and I must NOT fail". This mindset leaves us feeling small, and sometimes broken when life doesn't go our way.

When we are humble we gain self confidence, because we are no longer afraid of failure. With self-confidence we can firmly trust Divine Guidance. Filling up and filling out behaviors are no longer needed where confidence was once lacking. We stop engaging in unsustainable plans that result in temporary gratification, then exhaustion. i.e. Saying yes to an invitation, when you really wanted to say no. Staying in a relationship that is not fulfilling, because you are afraid to live alone. Starting a fad diet to lose weight, so that you will impress people that don't care about you. Eating an entire cake while upset, because you'd rather block the emotions arising, than feel them moving through you. Oh, the shit we will do to seek gratification, even if it's toxic. Yet, Maya Angelou reminds us, "We do better when we know better."

As we grow up into adults, it is our responsibility to reckon with our emotions as they come into our awareness. Much like a movie, the emotional body holds images of our past. **The primary reason the brain remembers the past is to better predict what will work in the future.** Please be kind to yourself as you listen and compassionately respond to the stories that keep you in pain. Try choosing a response from *your heart,* not a reaction from your childhood.

Part 4. Being Intentional

Stop wishing and make choices that set plans into action. Stop aspiring and start doing. Even if your beginning is messy, scary, or amateur--get going! Begin where you are. An intention is a goal with passion and purpose.

- Create Intentions
- Setting Goals
- Walk the Walk
- Drop Expectations

Create intentions

An intention is a mental impulse for your creative aim; seed energy for the goal. An intention is a thought casted outward-released. How can a seed grow while still sitting in your hand? Intentions may be cast several times a day. Whatever is burning in your soul, an intention gives it words, so that The Divine may give it wings. Hold these intentions in your mind and hands at your heart. Staying with these thoughts, kissing your hands and offering them up into the sky.

Meditation is a powerful way to harness your intentions. This opportunity to listen to your inner dialogue is like having a cup of tea with yourself. It is a time to sit with yourself and ask, **"How are you, sweetheart?"** The goal is not to judge, attach to, or resist what crops up. Just let it flow. If there are tears, let them come. Let it all come! Let it flow until you notice the spaces between the flow of emotion, thoughts, and memories. Let it all come and go like clouds in the sky. It is said that your highest Self is the sky, not the weather. In the spaces and gaps, you can sense the awareness of your true Self. You may tell yourself a story like you can't meditate, but is that true? How many times have you actually tried? You see, every time you sit quietly with the aim to meditate, *you are doing it!* Meditating isn't something you can touch. To a cerebral person, it may seem as if the mission was unaccomplished.

I grew up understanding how to pray (ask), but didn't understand mediation (listening) until I found Yoga in 2001. For me, it has made a positive difference in my life. My perceptions, attitude, compassion, and choices can shift COMPLETELY, if I sit with myself long enough to hear my heart's truth. If I am tense, I find it hard to sit for very long. Sometimes, I am not even aware of how tense, depressed, conflicted, or insecure I am feeling until I sit. Which in turn, tells me I *need* to sit longer! Yet still, there are stressful days I give myself permission to be where I am, and cut my time short, anyway.

Meditation is an opprotunity to give myself time and space to start the day off with an attitude of gratitude. Rushing out the door sets a hectic vibe for our day and swiftly leaves us feeling empty. Spending 5-30 minutes in a daily morning meditation is incredibly healthy. Try this:

Close your eyes and take a deep conscious breath through your nose and let it out your mouth. As you watch your thoughts, watch how your mind recalls memories. Watch how emotions arise to meet your mind. Allow this space. Sense your surroundings (sounds, scents). As this is happening, see if you can sense the Divine Observer. (The Mind that watches you watching yourself). This is the space to rest your whole heart. This is the space to cast your intentions and desires. This is the space to plant your desires. Then, with a single conscious exhale, detach from the intentions. Return to your breath. After resting with the Divine Observer, for as long as you can, open your eyes and write down in your journal what intentions you cast into God's deep soil.

Writing in our journal after meditation, helps us to recall our intentions. Your writings don't have to be short stories (although sometimes they can be lengthy and that is okay); they can be one sentence long. Whatever you need it to be, is what it will be. They may begin with words like: "help me, I will, and I must." Here's a few of my good and faithful intentions: "God, help me show up my best and highest Self today."

"Help me to pause long enough to ask myself, "What I am REALLY hungry for?" "I will go to the gym today and workout." "I must make time for Yoga today." Many people benefit from their own written affirmations, but there are other sources too. We have a plethora of beautifully written affirmations available to use in books and on social media. If sacred writings resonate with your path, they can be deeply nourishing as well. Whatever you choose, may it fill you up with love, not shame. If it doesn't fill your heart, it's not your path.

Try speaking an intention before raising your head from your pillow each morning. Our humanity anticipates we may weaken and something (or someone) might throw us off in the day. A morning intention can prepare us to respond from our highest Self. Without intention, impulses can overrule our better behaviors.

Intentions act as inner whispers rising to the surface when we need them to empower us. When we foster these inner whispers, they serve to remind our conscious mind of the path we have chosen. Intentions are most powerful when they come from a place of contentment, not desperation, lack, or need. Personal doubt and naysayers can unbalance us very easily. Remember to stay centered and refuse limiting beliefs.

Choose a methodology to create intentions. See if you can adopt one or more of the following ways:

1. Prayer and meditation
2. Keep a journal.
3. Use "post it notes" to remind you of your goals. Place them around your living spaces.
4. Speak aloud to yourself, "I want…I will…I can…."
5. Create a vision board every six to twelve months.

Setting Goals

Plan a life you would like to have. What do you want? What would be good for you? Why NOT go and get it? Discipline is a matter of disposition of order. Order is necessary, especially for those that are hopeless and nihilistic. Writing goals is like laying disciplinary structure on yourself to get chaos in check. Then you can move towards the state of liberation.

Personal Assessment 4:2

Writing monthly goals, quarterly goals, and annual goals are a plan to direct your aim toward the target. Document at least one monthly, quarterly, and annual goal using the **SMARTER** goal outline. The acronym SMARTER stands for: **Specific, Motivational, Accountable, Relevant, Touchable, Engaging, Responsible**. [3]

Your personal goals do not *have* to be specific to food, exercise or your body. Think more abstractly about thoughts and behaviors that play a role in fostering positive choices. Ask yourself...

Does my goal have meaning?

Does the meaning of my goal embody FINDING more meaning?

Is it emotionally charged?

Do I have the energy to carry it out?

Can my goal be tracked or accounted for?

How does this goal meet my needs?

What will I have as my final outcome?

Are my goal's processes able to hold my attention?

Is it worth my necessary time, energy and resources?

A quarterly goal example.

S (Specific) What is the goal, and can your goal be broken down into smaller steps?

I will increase my fruit and vegetable intake to four servings a day. I will purchase different fruits and vegetables each week to create variety. I will not be redundant in my choices for at least two weeks in a row. I will eat what I buy and be sure to place the food in my fridge where I can see it, as not to forget about them. I will pre-prep any veggies if possible (ex: chop cauliflower in advance) making my choice more convenient.

M (Motivational) Is this emotionally charged? Do you have the energy to carry it out?

I am motivated to be the healthiest I can be. I know I feel better when I eat enough plant foods. I can carry out this goal with ease and have the energy to make the effort to have more fruits and vegetables on hand.

A (Accountable) Can your goal be tracked or accounted for?

I will purchase enough to have at least two servings of each, daily. There will be none thrown away or uneaten at the end of the week. I will track my fruit and vegetable intake in my Evolve Healthy Food Diary.

R (Relevant) How does this goal meet your needs?

This goal is relevant, as I know body desires and thrives optimally on daily consumption of fruits and vegetables.

T (Touchable) What are the benefits of your outcome?

I will have more vibrant energy, increased mood, better bowel movements, aid in healing my gut and other physical aliments. Additionally, I can rest assured that I am taking the necessary step to preventing cancer, as science based evidence shows.

E (Engaging) Are the goal's processes able to hold your attention?

I will be engaged to do this because I will be entering the grocery store each week with a new technique to healthy shopping. It will cause me to think more strategically as I enter the produce section. It will open my eyes to other options and purchase enough fruit and veggies. I will explore fresh, frozen and dried options. I look forward to learning how to simplify my choices and make them a habit.

R (Responsible) Is it worth your necessary time, energy and resources?

Yes, my health is worth my time, energy and money!

Monthly SMARTER goals

Today's date _____

Projected outcomes by _____

S (Specific) *What is your goal? If possible, write concisely and break it down into smaller steps.*

M (Motivational) *Is it emotionally charged? Do you have the energy to carry it out?*

A (Accountable) *Can your goal be tracked or accounted for?*

R (Relevant) *How does this goal meet your needs?*

T (Touchable) *What will you have as your final outcome?*

E (Engaging) *Are the goal's processes able to hold your attention?*

R (Responsible) *Is it worth your necessary time, energy and resources?*

Quarterly SMARTER Goals

Today's date _____

Projected outcomes delivered by _____

S (Specific) *What is your goal? If possible, write concisely and break it down into smaller steps.*

M (Motivational) *Is the emotionally charged? Do you have the energy to carry it out?*

A (Accountable) *Can your goal be tracked or accounted for?*

R (Relevant) *How does this goal meet your needs?*

T (Touchable) *What will you have as your final outcome?*

E (Engaging) *Are the goal's processes able to hold your attention?*

R (Responsible) *Is it worth your necessary time, energy and resources?*

Annual SMARTER goals

Today's date _____

Projected outcomes delivered by _____

S (Specific) *What is your goal? If possible, write concisely and break it down into smaller steps.*

M (Motivational) *Is the emotionally charged? Do you have the energy to carry it out?*

A (Accountable) *Can your goal be tracked or accounted for?*

R (Relevant) *How does this goal meet your needs?*

T (Touchable) *What will you have as your final outcome?*

E (Engaging) *Are the goal's processes able to hold your attention?*

R (Responsible) *Is it worth your necessary time, energy and resources?*

Walk the Walk

Many of us know how to talk the talk. The knowledge for healthy living is available in many forms. However, those that walk the walk are the most influential. The most influencial health leaders aren't walking the walk with the hope others will *hear* them talk the talk. They do it because they want to strut their bodacious, high vibe energy, regardless of whether anyone notices or not. Others feel that, because human beings are a vibration! Your vibration can be so strong that others can *smell it* if you're genuine! We will attract what we are. No words are necessary when your energy is tuned in and turned on.

Many clients have asked me in the past for advice on changing their spouse, children, friends, etc. dietary habits. I have only one golden piece of advice for you: Walk the walk! Telling other what they "should do" carries no clout. Words do not matter much for those that aren't ready to hear them. Your actions are the master key. Others will see it, feel it, and perhaps even smell it! They will come to know it when they are ready, in *their* timing. The best thing you could ever do for those you hope to influence most is *be* the example.

Educate and share with others if they ask for your help. You will KNOW when it's a request. Better yet, you could clarify they are asking for your help. "**Are you asking me to share what I know works for me?**" If they are ready, they will usually respond with a simple, clear, wholehearted answer like, "Yes." What you say at that point can be very powerful, but it will never be as powerful as your walk!

 It's easy to talk the talk, but can you walk the walk?

Managing Expectations

Warning: Expectations can be the greatest source of disappointment. Expectations are often times an attempts to control the future. For best results write your goals in pencil, walk the walk, and manage expectations. Once we drop expectations we are allowing Divine Guidance to take the lead. Get out of the way and allow this creative process to weave its design through your hands! It is better to manage our expectations and enjoy our life with a few daily reminders:

1. **Get centered each day.** When centered, you are no longer dependent on your circumstances. The walk of your path that includes hills and valleys of the day, will not take you off your feet.

2. **Leave room for the unexpected to come.** Love what is, as it comes. When we try to direct our every detail of the day, we contract and miss many precious moments.

3. **Let go of controlling all expected outcomes!** The only thing we can control is how we respond to a given moment. Future outcomes are out of our control. Be grateful for this, because that is one hell of a responsibility.

4. **Take life a wee bit less seriously!** Life comes in and it goes out. It's like breathing in and out of your nose. In..and... Out. Life gives and takes away. Disappointment is natural. Remind yourself when feeling disappointed that you feel diss-appointment because you had expectations. As you continue doing your inner work, a new way of thinking and responding will arise. A better source of happiness exists. It lives within you. Let us not forget that some of the best gifts of life are the ones that come unexpectedly!

Personal Assessment 4:3

What are your expectations?

1. What expectations do you have about eating healthy?

2. What expectations do you have about the way your body could or should look?

3. Do either of these expectations above give you inner peace?

4. If not, what do they give you? If so, what does that inner peace feel like?

5. Can you drop the stressful expectations that make you feel disempowered? If not, why not?

6. Who would you be without expectations?

Part 5. Mindful Rituals

When we give ourselves the gift of daily sacred time, we are better equipped to show up at our best. With practice and remembrance that the work is never done, you can remain centered-even when life rolls out the hard knocks. Creating a mindful, daily ritual has one rule: it must be something you can do *every single day* that requires *no stressful* commuting. This sacred time should feel easy to slip into. Find a space within your home, or walking distance outside of your home. However, if the commute to get to and from this location isn't stressful or challenging to you, then commute on! For example, going to the gym may be a ritual for you, but a mindful daily ritual will also contain a few minutes of soulful introspection. Perhaps, the commute to the gym IS the ritual, afterall! Another example may be to enter the day gently, with a cup of coffee or tea and a meditation. Make your ritual convenient, simple and calming. If you only have five minutes, great! If you can make it one or more hours, good for you! It all counts, and every single second matters!

Rushing out the door most mornings sets a stressful tone for the entire day. When you're intentional about carving out sacred time in the mornings for yourself, the rest of your day will follow the energy you created. This may mean you wake up 10-60 minutes earlier each day, but I promise you, you'll have no regrets! Create your ritual, and be proactive on establishing boundaries surrounding it. If mornings are already saturated with things that are completed for others, some other appropriate time of the day *may* be in order. Remember, we must give to ourselves so that we may better serve others. Be kindly reminded that your ritual is just as important, if not more important, than the space you help to create in others lives, including your immediate family. Therefore, if that means getting up ten minutes earlier than usual, you are worth it! Be consistent with your valuable decision to take diligent care of yourself.

Mindful Ritual ideas.

1. Sit in prayer and meditation.
2. Prepare and eat a healthy breakfast.
3. Practice gentle yoga or create a stretch routine in the bed.
4. Walk your dog, leisurely or stroke your cat with your full presence.
5. Drink a tall glass of water and practice conscious breathing. (Prana)
6. Light a candle and sip coffee or tea.
7. Write or journal. Write 2-3 pages of stream of conscious thoughts.
8. Soak in a hot bath and listen to calm music.
9. Skin brush and moisturize.
10. Read sacred texts.
11. Knit/Crochet/Quilt
12. Doodle/Paint
13. Play an instrument.
14. Sing
15.Watch the sunrise or the sunset in silence.

What would you like to do for your mindful ritual?

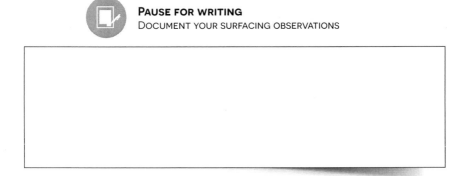

PAUSE FOR WRITING
DOCUMENT YOUR SURFACING OBSERVATIONS

Permission granted! Allow this mindful, daily ritual to be all about you—a sacred solo reflection event *all for yourself.* Having the company of another human being is not necessary during this time. Being a lover of my dog, I believe that pets are optional to include, because they are attached directly to the very part of us that we will be nurturing...our hearts!

Personal Assignment 4:4

Schedule an additional 10-60 minutes of time dedicated to your mindful ritual.

Design a plan for your day using clock time. Put in time for your family, work, commute, meals, mindful ritual, etc. Write in pencil. This may take a few tries.

- Bedtime _____
- 1-2 hours before bed (optional sacred time) __
- Last meal of the day _____
- Arrive home from work _____
- Commute time_____
- Work hours_____
- Breaks at work _____
- Arrive at work _____
- Commute time _____
- Dress for the day _____
- Mindful morning ritual _____
- Breakfast _____
- Awake time _____

Your Commitment

You now have direction to create a mindful ritual.

You now have a sensible, written blueprint that works within your needed time-frame.

 If you are ready to commit, read and sign this agreement:

I pledge to give myself permission to create and implement a mindful ritual for the entirety of this program.

Everyday, I will make this time for myself so that I will be ready to show up in life vibrating at my highest capacity: emotionally, physically, and spiritually.

I deserve to listen, tend to, and nurture myself with whole hearted care!

I will dedicate sacred time to myself each day.

_____

My Signature   Today's date

References

1. Brewer, Judson, MD, PhD. (2017). The Craving Mind: From Cigarettes to Smartphones to Love – Why We Get Hooked and How We Can Break Bad Habits. New Haven, CT: Yale University Press

2. Creative Commons Attribution-NonCommercial-ShareAlike 4.0 International License. Introduction to Physiology, 3.2. Our Brains Control Our Thoughts, Feelings, and Behavior. Retrieved from http://open.lib.umn.edu/intropsyc/chapter/3-2-our-brains-control-our-thoughts-feelings-and-behavior/

3. Mind Tools. (2018, March 25) Smart Goals: How to make your goals achievable.

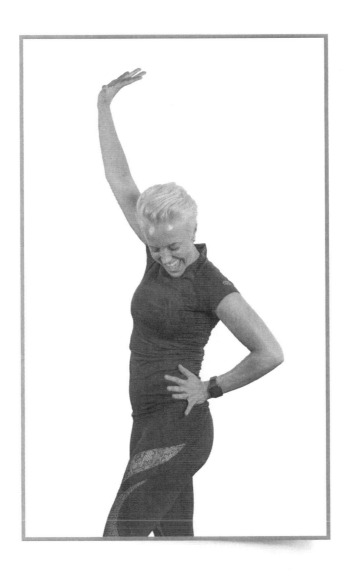

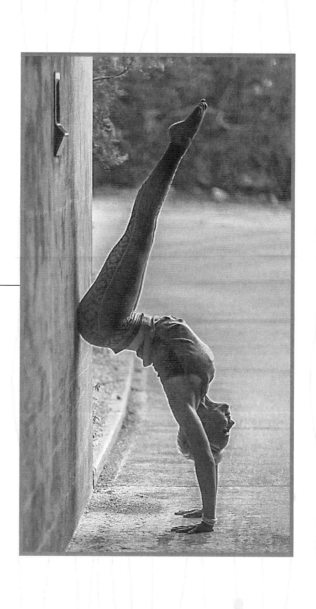

Phase V: Action

You can call it fitness, exercise, activity or movement, but like Nike says, "Just do it!" Without question, exercise provides positive outcomes. Take action! If your inner dialogue is, "I have to exercise", I challenge you to change your inner dialogue to, "I get to exercise." Your thoughts and words matter!

You can NOT be mentally or physically healthy without a routine. Pick a time to exercise and stick to it! Otherwise, you disregulate your circadian rhythms and they regulate your mood! Surround yourself with others that are taking action and have created healthy routines. Look around at your direct spehere of influence. Access and fix the things that announce themselves in need of repair. Perhaps, the greatest guilt you can experience is the sheer knowledge that you are not taking care of yourself. Are you leaving that responsibility to other people? If so, it is highly probable that you will be enveloped in guilt and shame, because you are not taking care of yourself, and thereby not living up to your full potential. There is a weight that resides on your shoulders if you choose to go along with that.

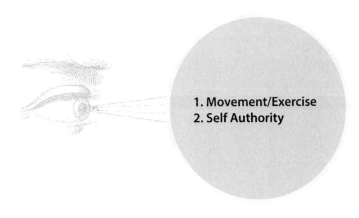

1. Movement/Exercise
2. Self Authority

Part 1. Movement/Exercise

Motivation to Exercise

Motivation requires a meaningful reason. What does exercise mean to you? What reason do you have to do it? Human beings become more alive in their minds and hearts when consciously moving their bodies. Ask yourself, "**What do I want my body to accomplish?**" Begin where you are; choose an activity that inspires a "I get to," instead of "I have to." If walking on the treadmill does not interest you, or causes you to cringe at the idea, don't choose the treadmill! If walking in your neighborhood invokes a peaceful mindset, do that instead!

What thoughts of fitness/exercise/activity/movement resonate with you? Consider the "get to" list below.

Check the reasons that resonate with you.

- ☐   I get to feel more alive
- ☐   I get to be stronger
- ☐   I get to resist depression
- ☐   I get to burn off old emotions (stored in my body)
- ☐   I get to flush my lymphatic system
- ☐   I get to reduce my risk for cancers
- ☐   I get to have good posture
- ☐   I get to be more clear-headed
- ☐   I get to become more grounded
- ☐   I get to generate more energy
- ☐   I get to feel good in my clothes
- ☐   I get to feel good naked

- ☐ I get to be a role model for my kids
- ☐ I get to lift my moods
- ☐ I get to correct the physical alignment that causes pain, and therefore reduce my chronic pain
- ☐ I get to reduce inflammation
- ☐ I get to strengthen my bones
- ☐ I get to take care of myself
- ☐ I get to reduce bloating
- ☐ I get to reduce pain
- ☐ I get to sleep better
- ☐ I get to age gently
- ☐ I get to improve my balance
- ☐ I get to improve my flexibility
- ☐ I get to de-stress
- ☐ I get to breathe easier
- ☐ I get to move more efficiently
- ☐ I get to boost my immunity
- ☐ I get to detox my body
- ☐ I get to attract healthy vibes
- ☐ I get to reduce health care cost
- ☐ I get to have skin that glows
- ☐ I get to enable healthy blood pressure
- ☐ I get to enable healthy cholesterol levels
- ☐ I get to have quality time in this body
- ☐ I get to prevent disease
- ☐ I get to decrease the symptoms of my current disease state

Personal Assessment 5:1

Choosing your mindset

Making time for conscious movement can seem like a challenge for many people. Affirming your reasons to exercise is a way to choose your mindset. Take a look again at the *get to* list on the prior page. Write down each sentence you checked on a sticky note. Hang the notes around your living spaces for at least one month. Whenever you see your note, read it out loud.

Choosing your type of activity

Movement is healthy for people of all shapes and sizes. Intensity and exercise choice will vary based on your body type, age, and the season in which you find yourself. High intensity exercise is not sustainable for most people their entire life. As a seasoned fitness professional, allow me to remind you that you do not have to "get after it" *every single workout!* Not everyone was designed to be an athlete, but we are most certainly designed to move! Movement is the master key to optimal physical health, *specifically*, proper resistance and cardiovascular training. Research shows that there are three important things to include in an ideal fitness prescription: resistance training, elevated heart rate, and movements that require sustained effort. If you workout just three times a week, you will benefit significantly. Ask yourself three questions: (I have written an *example* answer in parenthesis.) **What do I like to do that involves resistance training?** (weight lifting) **What do I like to do that raises my heart rate?** (cycle, versa climber) **What do I like to do that involves sustained effort?"** (Yoga) Embrace your answers, albeit they're conventional or eccentric. Whatever comes to your mind is a perfect place to start.

After consideration, document your three answers.
Be as specific as you can be about why you chose those things.

A lot of social media accounts tell us that we should be "killing it" at every workout; always rocking the ever elusive, six pack abdominals. *Sigh.* Not everybody is equipped to be (or even look) athletic— and THAT IS OKAY! Often, we only see the highlights of an athlete's high intensity workout and perceive it to mean only one thing-FULL THROTTLE, EVERY TIME! Workouts do not require continuous high intensity to obtain great health or a fine physique!

I started lifting weights when I was sixteen. I love everything about it. People often assume that my every workout is intense. Nope! Not all of my workouts (or seasons of workouts) have been "intense," but, they have definately been CONSISTANT. With experience and education, my knowledge of "smart" training has surpassed my need to "kill it" at every workout. I do not always feel like "going in and getting it," but, I "go in!" Understand?

If you are a competitive athlete with a commitment to high intensity training (monitored by professional strength coaches, athletic trainers, physical therapists, sports psychologists, and sports dietitians) then you are the exception, not the rule. If you fall within the majority of the population, choose activities that bring you pleasure. Choose activities that inspire you! Practicing the discipline of consistancy is enough. Do these to the best of your ability at least three times a week.

For optimal and personalized fitness programming, please consult with a seasoned, certified personal trainer or certified strength and conditioning specialist. Before you begin training, interview them. Ask to see their professional resume, credialing certificates, along with a list of past and present client references. There is an art to coaching and finding the right fit is worth your time and effort.

Choosing intensity

When selecting an intensity, consider choosing the energy you want to attract. What energy do you want to broadcast into your life? The physical vibration you emit is inpacting everything around you. You are contagious and your energy impacts mood. Your own mood, and everyone around you. Earlier, you created a list of your favorite activities. Ask yourself, **"How intense do I want to feel?"**

For those who may be overdoing intensity to the detriment of your body, I urge you to reconsider your exercise plan. When abundant stress (physical or emotional) is placed on your body for an extended amount of time, your body resists metabolic changes. There is such a thing as too much intensity and the body will contract when burnout occurs. Learn to tune in and ask the body how it's doing. The body speaks to us with its own language. The body can not lie. Below are three signs of exercise burnout.

Signs of Exercise Burnout

1. You have a fear of incorporating a rest day from exercise.

2. You think that if you are not pushing your body to the point of exhaustion at every workout, it's not worth exercising.

3. You are exercising for longer than 60 minutes per day and think you "have to" instead of "I get to."

Here is what you could do if you are experiencing signs of exercise burnout!

Yield!

Take 2-5 days off and rethink your motives. Seek out a fitness professional to help formulate a revised proactive plan that empowers sustainability.

You have reached exercise burnout when:

1. You have decreased performance

2. You have lost your gym mojo. "I get to" is instead, "I have to."

3. You are experiencing insomnia. You are having a hard time falling asleep or staying asleep.

4. Your resting heart rate has increased.

5. You feel sluggish throughout the day after your workouts.

6. Your appetite has diminished.

7. You are sore most of the time. Your delayed onset of muscle soreness (DOMS) never seems to go away.

Here is what you could do if you are experiencing any of the above signs.

Yield!

Take 7 days off and rethink your motives. Seek out a fitness professional to formulate a revised proactive plan that empowers sustainability.

Choosing your duration and frequency

Something is always better than nothing! If you have been sedentary for years, I invite you to shift your mindset and begin where you are! **Don't allow "all or none" thinking rob you of doing what you can each day. Work up to the following goals by increasing your time as your body becomes stronger.**

Most recently, the minimum amount of exercise recommended by the American Heart Association is 150 minutes per week of moderate exercise, or 75 minutes per week of vigorous exercise (or a combination of moderate and vigorous exercise). [1] You may break up those total minutes however you choose. Thirty minutes a day, five days a week is an easy format to remember. You may also divide your time into two or three segments of 10 -15 minutes per day, if you feel inclined. To reduce blood pressure or cholesterol, it is recommended that you elevate your heart rate for 40 minutes at a time, 3-4 times per week. This has undoubtedly shown to lower your risk for heart attack and stroke. Regardless of your choice in movement, select one that creates both joy and heat within your body. One of the simplest ways to effectively improve heart health is walking. It's free, easy, sustainable, and can be social.

If you are not new to exercise, include between 240-320 minutes per week of moderate to vigorous exercise. That equates to 40-55 minutes per day, 6 days a week. Remember, motion is lotion! Why not move your body six days a week? Include a rest day, as we all tend to need one day a week to just BE without DOING anything at all. However, if that's not for you, try 35-45 minutes a day, seven days a week. For OPTIMAL outcomes, invest 50-60 percent of your weekly exercise time in heavy lifting or other suitable forms of resistance training. These sessions may equate to 30-60 minute sessions, 1-3 times a week. Invest the other 40-50 percent of your exercise time in elevating your heart rate and other sustained efforts you are passionate about. These sessions may equate to 20-60 minute sessions, 1-6 times a week.

American Heart Association Recommendations (heart.org)

For overall Cardiovascular Health:
- At least 30 minutes of moderate intensity aerobic activity at least five days per week for a total of 150 minutes.

OR

- At least 25 minutes of vigorous aerobic activity at least three days per week for a total of 75 minutes; or a combination of moderate and vigorous intensity aerobic activity.

AND

- Moderate to high intensity muscle strengthening activity at least 2 days per week for additional health benefits.

For Lowering Blood Pressure and Cholesterol
- An average of 40 minutes of moderate to vigorous intensity aerobic activity 3-4 times per week.

Personal Assessment 5:2

Since Phase II, you have been planning your exercise days, type, and duration on your Proactive Plan worksheet. Traditional or nontraditional choices have been welcomed (and hopefully) embraced. I am hopeful that a smile comes from within when you think about, "getting to" exercise, instead of "having to!"

If you have been engaging in a routine and are ready to mix it up, this assessment is right on time! Discover and experiment with a new playful movement that comes from a place of enjoyment. For this week, add or exchange at least one of your typical workouts for a new activity. Creating variety invites new experiences, versatility, and metabolic changes.

Examples: Exchange roller blading/skating for walking. Introduce swimming and alternate it with your hiking days. Try a dance class instead of walking. Walk outside instead of on the treadmill. Take Pilates instead of lifting weights. Lift weights instead of Yoga. If none of these resonate with you, get creative! Shake it up and have fun!

What new activity will you try next week?

Part 2: Self Authority

Negative mental programming and negative environment are often responsible for lack of self-authority. You don't need anyone's permission to take care of yourself; you only need your own. It is important to know how to rule yourself! **The imperative of self authority is that you can never blame others!** That means placing boundaries around you and other people's thoughts, words and actions to move you to action. Use your own judgment and common sense. For example, you don't need a workout partner every time you exercise. Give yourself authority to do what needs to be done. This does not mean you do not engage in group fitness or other social forms of exercise. It just means that you have what it takes to get your workouts done, even when there is no one to be accountable to, besides yourself. When we have self-discipline, we gain the freedom to reach our fullest potenital. The more disciplined we become, the easier life gets. Perhaps this is because, when we practice self-discipline, we have the ability to overcome primal impulses. Acting on a whim (doing whatever we feel like doing) is a response to act out our subconscious programming to external situations.

The next time you find yourself wanting to skip your workout, inquire within before making the final decision to blow it off. For example, you decide you are not going for your morning strength training session when the alarm goes off. First, *notice* the impulse to choose against your commitment. Next, ask yourself at least two of these questions:

"What am I trying to accomplish?

"What do I want?"

"What am I resisting right now?"

"What is the emotion?"

"Will this decision be worth it to me at the end of this day?"

"Am I ignoring the truth, or am I facing it?"

"What do I feel like when I don't do it?"

"Is this my own choice?"

S Sweet Spot

It is time to honor our playful, primal instincts and feel good in our bodies! Close the shades, or not (ha!), and get naked! Turn on your favorite music and DANCE, wild and free. Erratic moves are encouraged! Humans have danced for centuries because it feels good and natural! We all move differently. If you believe there is a 'good' or 'bad' way to dance, it may be that you've adopted someone else's opinion. Opinions are not truth, so don't allow this story to govern or limit you. Dance however you want to!

Don't even try to skip this sweet spot! Yeah, you! If you are thinking of skipping this sweet spot, this sweet spot is ESPECIALLY for you! Liberate yourself! Step out of your comfort zone! Give yourself permission to become one with your body, one with the music and one with the universal mind!

Dance into and beyond the emotions that arise. You may laugh, scream, cry or even be super paranoid for a few minutes. It's all part of the experience! *Notice* how alive you become when you stop believing everything you think and JUST DANCE!

Dance, dance, dance! Dance, it changes everything. Shift your mood instantly! You are free! You've always been free, you just forget sometimes. I'm dancing right there with you, soul to soul! Let's go!

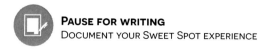

PAUSE FOR WRITING
DOCUMENT YOUR SWEET SPOT EXPERIENCE

References

1.   American Heart Association website. https://www.heart.org/en/healthy-living/fitness/fitness-basics/aha-recs-for-physical-activity-in-adults. Accessed August 4, 2018

Recommended resources for further fitness education:

- Z Health Performance Solutions—www.zhealtheducation.com

- National Strength and Conditioning Association—www.NSCA.com

- Keiser Fitness-- www.keiser.com

Reliable science-based fitness professionals on Instagram:

@coach_brettb
@strengthcoachtherapy
@drandygalpin
@gaithappens
@zhealth_performance
@physiomeetsscience
@dr.jacob.harden
@muscleandmotion

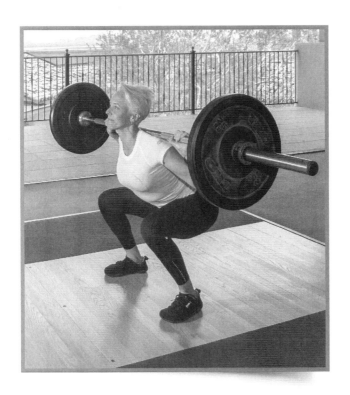

It takes courage to say yes to rest and play in a culture where exhaustion is seen as a status symbol.

-Brene Brown

Phase VI: Restoration

Restoration is a time to replenish what has been emptied. Author, Anne Lamott stated, "Almost everything will work again if you unplug it for a few minutes...including you." (Lamott, 2015) Restoration is action too! In this phase, we find ways promote our need to pause, get a good night's sleep, release stress, and explore creative outlets.

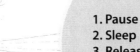

1. Pause
2. Sleep
3. Releasing Stress
4. Creative Outlets

Part 1. Pause

Pauses in your thinking can be used to stop intrusive, repetitive, self-defeating thoughts and move you into a new state of mind. When an unwanted thought comes to mind, say "pause" either silently or out loud. A physical reminder such as snapping an elastic band on the wrist, or body tapping may also be incorporated. An alternative technique is scheduling the intrusive thought for a particular time. For example, if you are disturbed by intrusive thoughts of self-defeat, you may pause and think, "I'll save those thoughts for a particular time each day." Inserting a pause, grants an opprotunity to manage or redirect intrusive thoughts. Another therapy technique is the *Miracle Question*. The miracle question, sometimes called the magic question, asks, **"If a miracle occurred that solved all of your problems, what would be different?"** This question emphasizes an action-oriented *pause*, that evokes a problem-solving mindset.

Intentions create our reality. How we perceive our life's experiences *is* our reality. Psychologists conclude that most of our perception comes from childhood and old belief systems.[1] When we believe our stressful thoughts, we can easily feel diminished. Twelve step programs use the phrase "stinking thinking," which is defined as a bad way of thinking. [2] Stinking thinking is believing you will fail and dreadful things are going to happen to you. Often, these fears aren't even things we can control. These thoughts require further self inquiry.

Personal Assessment 6.1

When we pause (wait), it saves us time next year. Pausing to listen (to ourselves and others), without reaction, promotes productivity. It makes us more efficient because we are more involved in the process of learning and gaining a deeper understanding. We can recognize things we want to remove from our plan or habit cycle, thereby instead, focusing our time on the things that work for us.

Book mark this page. Throughout the working of this Phase, write down the moments you were able to PAUSE. What was happening, and what pausing technique(s) did you find helpful in that moment?

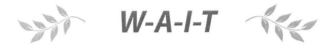

W-A-I-T

Why
Am
I
Talking?

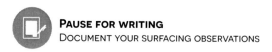

PAUSE FOR WRITING
DOCUMENT YOUR SURFACING OBSERVATIONS

A pause is like a crescent of time, unfolding the experience with intentional space around it. Be mindful—just because you learn to hit the pause button, doesn't mean it will always give you instant peace. However, pausing to observe what is real, along with a review of the details, may give you a deeper understanding of *your role*. Pausing can be a practice of discrimination. It may show up as a question like, "**Am I involved as a participant or an observer?**" By meeting ourselves with understanding, whether we are being approved or disapproved of (ourselves or others) ignites curiosity. Curoisity ignites learning, and learning is the opposite of surpression.

Organically, thinking happens. There is nothing you can do to stop it. Pausing doesn't mean withdrawing from reality. Non-responsiveness to avoid responding can be just as unhealthy as over-responding, i.e. talking too much. There are also times we don't know what to say because we are still trying to understand. If we need more information and it's okay to ask for it. Here are a few of my "go-to" questions that create a pause in a challenging conversation:

"I don't have enough information about this to answer right now. However, I do want to revisit this conversation."

"This does concern me, and I'd like to understand. Can you tell me more?"

"Can you say that differently so that I can try to understand your point of view better?"

Part 2: Sleep

A good night's sleep is one way to invest in your physical and mental health. Quality sleep increases your memory, immunity, metabolism, cellular repair, emotional processing (mental health) and learning ability. It also balances your body chemistry via hormones, and decreases the overall aging process.

Abundant evidence currently suggests that people who sleep for less than seven hours a night are more likely to become obese and develop Type 2 Diabetes. Supporting research states that sleep deprived adults have altered appetite hormones. These unbalanced hormones make you feel hungrier and less satiated throughout the day. Adults that are sleep deprived often crave sweet foods. [3] An average of 300 extra calories are consumed the following day after a poor night's rest. A few nights like this and you can quickly see how it can impact your health and body composition.

Good sleep hygiene, such as having a regular bedtime each night, results in decreased cortisol (the hormone that wakes you up) and an increased melatonin (the hormone that makes you sleepy). If you stay up late (more than one hour beyond your usual bedtime) your body produces more cortisol. The increase of cortisol before bed influences a release of stored glucose (blood sugar) from your muscles or liver. When there is too much glucose swimming inside the blood stream while you sleep, whether you are diabetic or not, the body cannot rest optimally, burn body fat as readily, or release abundant growth hormone (the fountain of youth hormone). [4]

According to the National Sleep Foundation, over one third of people in the United States say that their sleep quality is poor. Although, it is difficult to measure sleep quality because of its "subjective experience," the National Sleep Foundation agrees on a few metric questions that contribute to good sleep qualities for adults. [5]

Good sleepers will answer "Yes" to at least two of these questions.

1. Do you fall asleep in thirty minutes or less?

2. If you wake up, do you stay awake for less than five minutes, once per night?

3. Are you asleep eighty-five percent or more of your total sleep hours each night? (That's approximately less than twenty minutes of wake time during the night)

Poor sleepers will answer "Yes" to at least two of these questions.

1. Does it take you more than one hour to fall asleep?

2. Do you wake up in the night on four or more occasions?

3. Are you awake for forty minutes or more during the night?

DNA controls bodily rhythms in many ways. Our bodies don't run on one clock, but many; they are built into the cell's genetic programming. The master rhythm that sets all the others appears to be sleep. Without a good night's sleep, brain activity and hormonal balances are quickly thrown off, and conditions that seem far removed from sleep, such as obesity, are worsened. Sleep is also a major reducer of stress. When it comes to sleep, quality and quantity matter. The adult human being needs 7-9 hours of sleep every twenty-four hours. How you feel each day hinges on how many hours of sleep you had the night before, and is of equal importance to managing your stress, dietary and exercise choices. [6] If you are feeling fatigue during the day (even following the *Evolve Healthy* nutrition blueprint, and getting enough movement) it may be time to explore getting back to your body's natural circadian rhythm. Many people have challenges falling asleep, staying asleep, and waking up once asleep.

We will awaken more refreshed and energized when keeping a regular sleep-wake schedule, in lieu of tracking the total number of hours slept. For example, If I go to bed every night at 10 p.m. and wake every morning at 7 a.m., regardless if on a weekday or weekend, my body will most likely feel optimal. If I get nine hours of sleep (based on the time I hit the sack and wake the next day) I don't always wake feeling refreshed and optimized.

I admit, I'm like a koala bear and love my sleep time. I am a long sleeper and dream a lot. I do believe this is genetic. My body prefers at least nine hours of uninterrupted sleep. I used to fight this biological need for nine hours, until I realized through my research that it's natural for some to need more sleep. I recognized from my own struggles, and working with clients over the years, that changing sleep patterns are not easy at first. For best results, pick a time to go to bed and wake up each day. Stick to it, regardless of whether you have to be somewhere in the morning or not.

Consider the following suggested sleep strategies for a good night's sleep. I have compiled these strategies from reserach, and alternative health care professionals that I have worked with in the past. Try one at a time for seven days to collect data. Stay the course as you explore, then adopt, an effective sleep ritual.

Strategy #1. Find your rhythm

To determine how many hours you need of sleep each night, set a time to go to bed and wake up for the week, experimenting with seven, eight and nine hours of sleep. If you set aside seven sleep hours and notice you don't want to get out of the bed for three days in a row, try setting your sleep time to eight hours for the next three days. Perhaps, you are like me and need nine hours. Let it be so. Yes, this may mean you watch less or no television in the later evenings. Feeling "high-vibe" each day is worth the sacrifice. Be sure to calculate your bedtime. (When you normally feel tired and naturally desire to recline.) P.S. This is the time the average American begins watching television at night.

If you need to rest more, consider a daytime nap as an alternative to sleeping in. The more often you sleep in, the more fatigued you may be from disrupting your normal rhythm. Consider calculating a wake time that allows for a mindful daily ritual. I highly recommend you ditch the siren-like alarm clock sound to wake up. Instead, try soothing, zen-like sounds. They are a more peaceful and natural way to awaken. It is said that if you need an alarm clock to wake up, what you really need is an earlier bedtime, although I have found I STILL need an alarm. Honor your needs.

Strategy #2. Nap if you need to

Although napping can help you rejuvenate, biologically, it cannot make up for a full night's sleep. If you need a nap, and you can make the time for it, "Go for it!" If possible, limit your naps to 20-60 minutes.

Strategy #3. Create mood lighting

Melatonin is a naturally occurring human hormone in your that is reactive to light and regulates your sleep-wake cycle. No supplement necessary! We can use this built in hormone to our advantage to help us get sleepy and stay asleep too.

During the day, expose yourself to as much sunlight as possible. Begin your day with 100% sunlight, even if it's through the windows. Pull your shades up as soon as your feet hit the floor. Let as much sunlight into your home and workspace as possible. Create a work space closer to the window. Get outside in the sunlight and fresh air as often as you can each day. Even if it's for five minutes here and there, it counts! If you live in a grey climate and are having sleep challenges, invest in a light therapy box for greater light exposure.

During the night, avoid lighted screens one to two hours before bed. Blue light emitting from your phone, tablet, computer, and television interfer with the release of melatonin. If you had the thought, "And miss my shows?", then consider viewing them at an earlier time of the day.

Saying no to late night television will help you gain a relaxing slumber. You can also lower the light setting on your devices, invest in light altering software or blue screen filter eyewear. Consider reading or listening to audiobooks (or music) instead.

About two hours before your bedtime, set some mood lighting. Dim the lights throughout your living space to help facilitate an increase in melatonin and a decrease in cortisol. Make use of candles, dimmer switches and low wattage bulbs instead of overhead lighting. When it's time to get into bed, make sure the room is as dark as it can be. If you get up in the night, limit how much light you turn on, and think again before getting on any electronic devices. The light will affect your melatonin levels within a couple of minutes. Night lights in the nearby hallway or bathroom are fine but keep the space in your bedroom as dark as possible. If this is impossible, consider using a night mask or blackout shades.

Strategy #4. Exercise Timing

If possible, limit intense exercise to no less than three hours before bed. When we exercise we speed our metabolism, elevate body temperature and stimulate hormones, such as cortisol. Cortisol is not a bad thing, however, increasing it at night can affect how well we sleep. Cortisol is what wakes us up in the morning. On the contrary, low-impact exercises such as an evening stroll, gentle yoga, or stretching does aid in relaxation by decreasing cortisol and increasing melatonin.

Strategy #5. Food and Drink Timing

Daily consumption of complex carbohydrates, lean proteins, heart healthy fats, and fresh herbs help promote good sleep. Ideally, dinner time will occur no later than two hours before bed. This will give your body time to metabolize the food you ingest so that you are not working on churning food while your body is sleeping. This will also allow growth hormone to work its magic while you sleep.

Limit the consumption of caffeine after high noon if you are sensitive to it. For many, caffeine can affect sleep rhythms if consumed 10-12 hours before bed. Limit or cut out alcohol in the evenings. While you may feel a night cap brings you greater relaxation, research shows that it is interfering with your sleep cycle. Limit any other large quantity of hydrating beverages right before bed, as the need to urinate can contribute to interrupted sleep.

Strategy #6. Create a sleep sanctuary

Do your best to limit noise; earplugs, white noise or box fans may be in order. If you share a bed, and your partner has bedtime vices (television, tablets or computer) and is not on board with a new sleep routine, invest in a pair of headphones and request that they use them while you sleep. A night mask may be necessary to block light from the television. A white noise machine or box fan is a practical option for those that are noise sensitive. White noise machines and box fans can snuff out noises such as barking dogs in the distance, traffic, or another person's audible breathing in the other room. Keeping your bedroom at a cool 65°F or 18°C will enhance your ability to stay asleep. Invest in a good mattress, foam toppers, quality sheets, covers, and pillows! Be picky about your pillow support- your head and neck deserve the attention. Ensure the bedding allows for movement without getting tangled. Make it a habit to wash your sheets once a week; clean sheets on the bed are a fine dessert to the end of a productive day!

Limit working on your computer, watching television or surfing the internet in the bedroom. Create a sacred space that is strictly for sleeping and intimacy *only*. Decorate it with beautiful things. Choose room scents and colors that make you feel relaxed and sensual. Consider limiting photographs of other people in your bedroom, excluding ones of yourself and your lover.

S Sweet Spot

Create a bedtime ritual this week. Which sleep strategies do you want to try to deepen your relationship with sleep? Spend a moment contemplating your bedroom. Is it time to buy new bedding? Do you need to unclutter your sleep sanctuary? What can you do to your bedroom that would create alluring slumber? Invest in your space and rekindle your love affair with sleep.

Part 3: Releasing Stress

Breathwork

In Latin, the word breath means 'spiritum', or 'spirit.' [7] To consciously breathe, we can practice belly breathing through deeper inhales and exhales. Shallow breathing is generated from the throat or chest. Placing your mind on your breath is a practice that energizes and fuels the body. Its creates a mind and body stillness that prepares you for relaxation and immediate stress release. Try it on! Discover a form of restoration that can be obtained anywhere you are.

Below are two examples of introductory breath work. You might also learn useful techniques at a Yoga, Tai Chi or Qi Gong class. These practical methods come highly recommended, especially in moments of stress or panic. They can be done in the midst of an unpleasant conversation or driving in crazy traffic.

Breathing to the Count of Four

- Inhale through your nose to the very slow count of four. 1, 2, 3, 4.
- Aim to fill the entire chest cavity with air-rib cage and diaphragm.
- At the top of the inhale, at the count of 4, just when you think you cannot inhale anymore, sip that little bit more in.
- Relish (hold) at the top of the breath for a count of four. 1, 2, 3, 4. Focus more here and feel the stillness inside.
- Exhale through your nose to an even slower count of four. 1, 2, 3, 4.
- At the bottom of the exhale, at the count of 4, just when you think you cannot push anymore air out, huff that little bit more out.
- Relish (hold) at the bottom of the breath for a count of four. 1, 2, 3, 4. Focus more here and feel the stillness inside.
- Repeat for at least 5 sets.

Breathing to the count of four is an easy and powerful technique. You may experience burning in your lungs at first. But very soon into your practice, breaths will become stronger and deeper. The count of four breaths may become five or six. The focus of where to inhale and exhale can move all over the body. For example, you may focus on breathing through the soles of your feet and out the crown of your head. Or, breathing in through your heart and out through your fingertips. Wherever you want to focus your attention, let it be so. There is no wrong way to consciously breathe.

To generate heat in your body, try ocean breathing.

Ocean Breath (Ujjayi Pranayama)

- Inhale long and deep through your nose, with mouth closed, directing the breath to the back of your throat.
- Exhale a long and slow breath through your nose, with mouth closed. As you exhale, place the tongue on the roof of your mouth as you constrict the muscles in the back of your throat. This will create a thin and long exhale that sounds like a hissing, or ocean waves crashing on the shore in the distance.
- Repeat for 3-10 minutes. As your mind wanders, bring it back with a gentle focus on your ocean breath.

For clarity and demonstration, search YouTube for these breathing techniques, along with other techniques such as, breath of fire and single nostril breath. [8, 9] Whatever breathing technique resonates with you is worth practicing on a regular basis for stress release.

Stretching

Stretching promotes well-being and restoration. In my opinion, the greatest part about stretching is that it requires no fancy equipment, and it can be done most any place (including the comfort of your home.) Here are a few exceptional reasons to stretch each day.

1. Decreases risk for injuries. Stretching increases your range of motion and allows your body to flow in life instead of being too rigid. When our body is rigid, something as simple as stepping off curbs can cause you to pull a muscle.

2. Improves posture. When you improve muscular balance, your posture improves by allowing muscles to hold you upright. Stretching helps create alignment and balance, allowing your muscles to work in harmony, instead of fighting antagonistic strain in one area versus the other.

3. Reduce low back pain. Americans are "flexion addicts". Flexion occurs at the hips when you are in a seated position. We sit to work, eat, drive, write, read and more. Because we sit so often, we have shortened and less mobile hamstrings, hip flexors, and quadriceps. These shortened muscles can create a tilt in your hips which pulls on your back muscles, ultimately leaving you with aches or pain.

4. Increases blood flow to soft tissues. This one is very simple. Much like exercise, increased blood flow means more oxygen-rich blood is carried through your body, creating ALIVENESS! It also means nutrients received through food are more readily

absorbed. Joint synovial fluids increase as blood flow increases, thus creating greater range of motion, less joint pain, and a reduced risk for joint degeneration.

5.   Quiets the mind. Stretching and Yoga brings you back into your body. Sometimes this is very restorative and relaxing; other times it is emotional. Whatever the practice brings you each day, let it flow. The beauty and the terror of getting in your body may guide you to personal revelations.

I seek stretching opportunities everywhere. Objects call out to me as if to say, "Lean here, fold over me, step this way." The door jams, the wall, the yoga mat, the weight bench, the kitchen chair, the office chair, and the grocery store cart, to name a few unconventional objects. Don't forget the good ol' floor too! Some days you may be inspired to stretch for five minutes, others you may carve out 30-60 minutes. Whatever the duration, your body loves every moment of it! Remember not to force yourself into any positions with brute strength. If you can't breathe (at all) in the stretch, you shouldn't be in it.

S Sweet Spot

Stretch for at least ten minutes. You can do a "here and there" approach. If dedicating some floor time doesn't seem like your cup of tea, Take a yoga or stretch class to learn some new moves. Taking a class, even if inconsistently, increases your home stretch toolbox; a "go to" set of stretches for daily needs.

Prayer & Meditation

As discussed in Phase IV, regular mediation is worth exploring. Researchers continue to study the health benefits of meditation. Meditation increases body awareness by reshaping our brains with positive chemical activity at a genetic level, according to neuroscientists. Not only does it promote creative thinking, it reduces anxiety by allowing our brain to de-stress from the nervous system. Focus, multitasking, and enjoyment of mundane everyday tasks (like making your bed) increases with a regular meditation practice. Additionally, relationships improve, because meditation enhances connection and acceptance of others. It returns you to The Source—Love. Meditation changes your entire energy vibration. As alpha brain waves increase in your brain, they radiate all through your body, affecting your entire energy field far beyond what you might imagine. [10]

If you are new to meditation, and you'd like more guidance on how to meditate, I recommend the books, *True Refuge* by Tara Brach, PhD, *The Universe Has Your Back* by Gabrielle Bernstein, and *A Mind At Home With Itself* by Byron Katie. If you prefer electronic availability, check out Headspace.com. This digital platform offers "bite-sized guided meditations for a busy lifestyle."

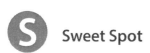 Sweet Spot

Take five minutes at lunchtime to sit alone with eyes closed. This can be done before or after you eat. Do nothing more than literally, close your eyes, sit with your best posture, and breathe. If you need to focus on something, affirm what you are doing and repeat these three words, "Rest, reset, and digest." Set a timer for five minutes. You may be surprised to find that a five-minute meditation will fly by and leave you feeling as if you just took a power nap.

Part 4: Creative Outlets

Creative outlets, such as painting, doodling, crafts, dance, music, writing, gardening, knitting, tiling, and landscaping, allow us to express ourselves and birth creative things. When we allow ourselves to really go for it without inhibition, dismissing our inner critic that whispers, "You're not creative," "You're not going to be good enough at that," "You'll screw it up," or "You're doing it wrong," we finally have the opportunity to discover that we *do* have creative abilities. Each creative ability looks different and don't you dare compare yours to ANYONE ELSE! This includes your past self. Ask yourself, **"What do I want to create?"** Perhaps, you will be naturally skilled and find awe in your ability. Or, you could find that you simply enjoy the process. Over time, if you are dedicated to the process in any varying degree, you will enhance your skill set, organically. Either way, creative outlets are not about winning a golden goodie at a competition. They are about allowing your inner light to shine.

Music

Music can shift mood quickly. Music can intoxicate your spirit. The power of a song's tempo, melody, harmony, and lyrics can shift your outlook almost immediately. Think about what music you are listening to currently. What theme is on your playlist? What is the message you continue to hear in your music each day?

When I moved back to Alabama, after being away for many years, my natural desire was to get in the mood with some country music as I drove down country roads. At first, it was great. I was singing along about the simple life, sweet tea and mama. It's okay to laugh, I am laughing too! Anyway, there were songs about breaking up, making up and creating drama in a supposed, "loving relationship". After a couple of weeks, I realized that a part of me was becoming identified with their message. I felt sad after listening to these songs and I even noticed I was taking on a victim persona in my own relationships.

My awareness was all it took; that reality check catapulted me to ask, **"Is this my story or theirs?"** From this, I was clear it wasn't what I wanted to be singing every day. I certainly didn't want to feel sad or be the victimized woman. Getting intentional about what music floods your energy field *is* important.

No, country music is not bad and will not make you a sad person. The moral of this story is that music shifts our moods. Choose music that does not increase confusion, anxiety, or sadness. **A confused, fearful, anxious and sad mind is out of balance.** Get proactive and invite music to elevate your spirit. Create a few playlists around desired moods. Consider the following moods:

- Joyful & Exuberant
- Grateful
- Gentle & Kind
- Loving
- Peaceful

Singing! Sing whether you have a beautiful voice or not! Just sing! Singing clears your throat. The throat is the energy center of the body that is about your inner truths and clear communication. Ask yourself,, **"What is it that I need to say that I am not saying?"** Singing can help clear the way. Think of this practice as a gateway to the spoken and the unspoken. Singing can release the desires of your heart. Be intentional with your songs of choice. Sing wherever you feel inspired to sing! Open your mouth and let it come into this world! Sing in the shower, car, into the mirror, or even on a stage in a karaoke joint. It's all such good medicine.

Have you been wanting to try vocal lessons? Now is the time! Thought about joining a choir? Go sign up! If the thought of singing as a stress release feels completely foreign and ridiculous then consider, at the very least, clearing your throat by screaming into a pillow. It is NOT overrated!

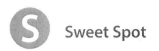

Sweet Spot

Create two music playlists. One for stress release, and one for uplifting joy. Be intentional about *how you want to feel* as you contemplate each song's rhythm, melody and lyrics.

Art

Painting, drawing, and crafting have a way of bringing our attention into the present moment. It is hard to think of much else while creating art. Coloring books, paint by number and doodling count too! For many artists I know, art is a stress reliever. Are you an artist? Do you aspire to be one? Stop aspiring and start doing! Some people do not even realize they have creative gifts until they finally try it. I was one of those people. For most of my life, I would say, "I can't paint or draw, but my brother can." My brother was known as the artist in my family. We all praised him for his talent and this became his identity to me-"My brother the artist". I never even tried painting or sketching, because it never crossed my mind. I was okay with my story that he was the only one in the family that could have this talent. That my gifts were elsewhere. While living in Sedona, Arizona, a very artsy town, I saw a sign for a beginner painting class. I had the thought for the first time, "What if I have the ability to paint? Could it be genetic?" Not minding if it turned out to be a terrible idea, I enrolled in my first painting class. It was an insightful reckoning. Wait! I'm not saying I was amazing, but I did see potential. I have painted six pieces since that first class.

I paint for fun and to move energy through me. In fact, painting while writing this book was a strategy for those times I needed discipline to write for a block of time. Between thoughts (or my need for a cerebral break) I would paint. I set up my canvas on an easel, paint for a few minutes, then return to writing when I felt ready. I share my paint story to encourage those of you reading this who have already thought that this particular outlet isn't for you.

If you've never tried, I dare you to try! If you have tried before, perhaps when you were younger, try it again! Who knows? You may have a different perspective about the process, enabling an artistic edge. You may discover that you have an amazing gift! At the very least, you will create unique decor for your home, or gifts for others. Enjoy yourself as you explore this creative outlet. It may be just what you've been looking for to help you decompress.

Service

What if the smallest thing you've done for others occupies a large part of their heart? Giving and receiving are seeds of the soul and merciful stress busters! The gift is indeed in giving. This is the true meaning of service. When you make a contribution to a person, act or cause, you are making a difference, whether it is recognized or not. By doing deeds, big or small, you are spreading love and compassion into this world. Your competence and self-confidence naturally spread to other aspects of your life: relationships, work, and life goals. Being in service, you feel a sense of purpose. This purpose then offers a stronger appreciation for those that care about the things you care about too.

The wellness benefits of helping others and pouring into causes that matter to you is radical! People who involve themselves in service have better mental and physical health than those who do not. Social interaction builds commitment and interest, both of which decrease depression. Service work takes your thoughts away from yourself (and your problems) and focuses them towards helping others. It may lessen your worry or depressing thoughts, as well as increase your self-esteem. Often, volunteers recieve as many benefits (or more) as those they are helping. Purpose, thought and body movement are ingredients for the brain's release of dopamine; the happiness hormone. What are you passionate about and how can you be of service?

Whether you're a parent, a career professional, or a volunteer in your community, *you are in service*. Additionally, consider small deeds as they present themselves throughout your day. When you see some trash on the side of the road during your walk, pick it up. When you notice an elderly person struggling to open the door, assist them. When you notice your spouse zooming through the house to complete a task, ask them, "How can I help?" I challenge you to find micro-service tasks each day. **See a need and fill it**. Discover the mental and physical effects of being in service.

Community service ideas:

- Mentoring
- Museums
- Food Banks
- Community Gardens
- Environmental Clean Up
- Soup Kitchens
- Local Events for a Cause
- Local Athletics
- Hospital
- Nursing Homes
- Hospice Visitation
- Library Readings
- Animal Rescues
- Animal Adoption Centers
- Homeless Shelters
- Art Show support
- Struggling Local business

Other

There is no such thing as one size fits all when it comes to creativity.

Here are a few other ideas of creative outlets to express yourself:

- pottery
- party planning
- sculpting
- knitting, sewing, stitching
- interior designing
- tile work
- hairstyles, tattoos, piercings
- treasure hunting at thrift stores
- antiquing
- writing
- landscaping
- wood working
- furniture upcycling
- cooking

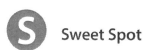 **Sweet Spot**

Try your hand at painting or drawing! Purchase a canvas, doodle notebook, or enroll in a creative class. Have zero expectations on the outcome. Simply give way to an experience with art, however it moves through you.

Or

Investigate how you might become involved in a community service or other creative outlets. Go enjoy yourself! Afterwards, write about your experience on the next page.

References

1. Sisgold, S. (2013, June 4). *Psychology Today.* "Limiting Beliefs" Retrieved from https://www.psychologytoday.com/us/blog/life-in-body/201306/limited-beliefs

2. Hunt, R. (2014, May 13). Transcend, A Recovery Community."Alcoholism: Stinking Thinking Leads to Drinking". Retrieved from https://transcendrecovery-community.com/alcoholism-stinking-thinking-leads-to-drinking/

3. Greer, S. M., Goldstein, A. N., & Walker, M. P. (2013). "The impact of sleep deprivation on food desire in the human brain" Nature Communications, 4, 2259. http://doi.org/10.1038/ncomms3259

4. Hersch, E. C., & Merriam, G. R. (2008). "Growth hormone (GH)–releasing hormone and GH secretagogues in normal aging: Fountain of Youth or Pool of Tantalus?" Clinical Interventions in Aging, 3(1), 121–129.

5. Hewings, Martin PhD, Y. (2018, May 17). "Determining the Quality of Your Sleep" [Nexalin Blog]. Retreived from https://nexalin.com/determining-the-quality-of-your-sleep/

6. Van der Helm, E., Gujar, N., & Walker, M. P. (2010). "Sleep Deprivation Impairs the Accurate Recognition of Human Emotions" Sleep, 33(3), 335–342.

7. Merriam-Webster. *Spirit.* (2018, May 1). Retrieved from https://en.wikipedia.org/wiki/Spirit

8. Gia Meditation. (2014, March 21). *Nadi Shodhana Pranayama* "Alternate Nostril Breathing (Tutorial)" Retrieved from https://www.youtube.com/watch?v=3E_-M-3Mt9c

9. Baer, Geoffery. (2007, August 6). "Kundalini Yoga Breath of Fire Primer" Retrieved from https://www.youtube.com/watch?v=zedVvFEh1ck

10. Bergland, C. (2015, April 17). *Psychology Today.* "Alpha Brain Waves Boost Creativity and Reduce Depression" Retrieved from https://www.psychologytoday.com/us/blog/the-athletes-way/201504/alpha-brain-waves-boost-creativity-and-reduce-depression

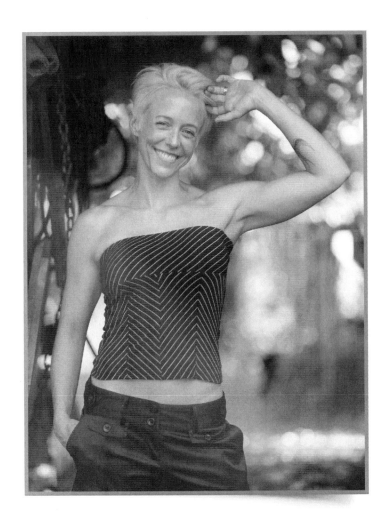

Rock bottom will teach you lessons that mountain tops never will.

-Author Unknown

Phase VII: Reflection

Reflection is contemplating where you've been and where you are now. Through contemplation, and living in the hard questions, we intrinsically connect to The Source. In this final phase of *Evolve Healthy,* you will be challenged to reflect on your *current* relationship with food, body image, and the practice of gratitude. Phase VII is inspired to highlight your journey and write your story.

Reflection requires self-examination. It happens when we take time to be introspective and review our life journey so far, to ponder our lessons, and to think about what is most important to share. Sharing our thoughts, perceptions and feelings, as there are others that want to know what was most important in our lives, and to learn from both the good and difficult life experiences. It is because I reflected on my journey that this book is a thing in the world! I am not saying you have to write a book, or even share what you write with others, but it may turn out to be the most LIBERATING of all *Sweet Spots* yet.

Inquiry works best when you quit trying to find definite answers and begin writing. In doing so, you are able to let go of resistance, and ride the waves of your story. We hit crests and troughs, weather storms, and enjoy the calm evenings when the waves are low. You are on an endless wave in the ocean, sometimes at the crest and other times in the trough of the wave. We are all in the ocean together.

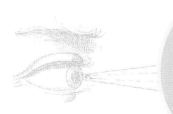

1. Food Liberation
2. Body Image
3. Gratitude
4. Paying it Forward

Part 1. Food Liberation

One of my favorite authors, Brene Brown said, "When you deny the story, it owns you. When you own the story, you get to write the ending." [1]

Food liberation is psychological. The "Thinker" (logical you), and the "Feeler" (emotional you) both experience food. The experience of eating food, thinking, and feeling are all wrapped together-they are all one. If you try to stabilize one without the other (anxiety likes to separate our experiences) you will find yourself in conflict.

There are a multitude of approaches to eating a healthy diet. However, there is no perfect approach to food. The science of nutrition is constantly proving and disproving itself—we are always learning more about foods and the way we eat. I believe relativity is the true constant. Continue to ask yourself, **"Which food concept feels most practical and sustainable for me, right now?"**

Food serves as a universal communication, and most of us enjoy it. It comes naturally; intuitively. Every day we think about food at some point. Our geographic food culture and our individual emotional connection to food, play a large part in our perception of food.

When you make up your mind and begin working to unveil your emotional triggers, your internalized stories from childhood, and continue the quest of self examination on how you use food to fill up the void in your life, food will lose its power over you. One day at time, you will learn to accept food for fuel AND pleasure making choices (such as enjoying more or less sugar) will have less bearing on how you feel about that choice. Abstinence works for some, and doesn't work for others. Adopting moderation gives the moderate tempermented, disordered eater, permission to "eat the cookie," mindfully. Intuitive eating is an invitation to enjoy food without shame or guilt.

You'll notice that you do not have to "should" on yourself to eat healthy. You may delight to discover over time that enjoyment of eating healthier food becomes easier. As your food relationship evolves, you begin including all types of foods, none of which feels like punishment. I promise this is possible.

Food liberation grows when you love and accept YOURSELF, and the food experience *as it is*. Negative emotions about yourself, food, and eating take time to heal. Having the courage to own (and share) the story you are telling yourself is a powerful way to heal.

Since Phase III, you have documented your food intake, the emotions present, and where you felt them in your body while eating. In doing so, the observation of your thoughts has made you different. How much different? Let's explore.

Food liberation is also about forgiving yourself. If you are ready to connect, forgive and accept your story, embrace this next personal assessment, wholeheartedly. Writing gives a voice to that which cannot (or will not) be silenced. When we choose to write, it helps us work things out. From working it out, we share our process and its raw, beautiful vulnerability. Often times our stories inspire others to lean into their own personal process. The previous writing assessments you have completed have prepared you for this assessment. Today is the day you begin writing *your* FOOD LIBERATION story!

Personal Assessment 7:1

What is your relationship with food? Examine your past motivations. Look closely. Consider the following questions as you write. Allow the thoughts to come to you. No matter how much they hurt, or how many tears fall out of your eyes, don't resist them. Keep the pencil moving, even if in between thoughts. Do not worry about proper grammar or spelling. Be brave as you allow your internal dialogue to release.

- What does food mean to you?
- How does food make you feel?
- When did this food relationship begin? How old where you?
- What was the story you told yourself about food?
- Who told you that story? Was it you or someone else?
- How did my intentions about eating (or not eating) produce the experiences I had?
- How have my intentions about eating (or not eating) produced the experiences I am having now?
- What is my *real* intention for food liberation?
- What would food liberation look like in your life? What is an ideal relationship between you and food?
- How would you show up in life differently if you were food liberated? Give 2-3 examples.

Take a deep breath. Sweetheart, sometimes you don't have the answers right away. If you don't have them yet, don't force them. When I ask my spiritual warrior friends hard questions, I wipe my brow with relief when they reply, "I don't have that answer, D." That honest and blunt comment reminds me that we cannot know everything, nor do we need to. Through the unknown, we learn how to trust the process or resist it. A sincere, "I don't know," feels way more like human connection to me than someone's regurgitated dogma or socially conditioned, classical education. The humility it takes to hear another intelligent person utter, "I don't know," is music to my ears. You're not alone, we don't know everything either. **If you don't know, try living in the questions** until the answers come.

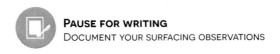
Congratulations, you have set universal order to your ideal relationship with food. Revisit your written story at least once a week. You will soon find your ideal summary unfolding. There is nothing more to do. Liberation does not come from pleasure seeking or trying harder. It comes from practicing self awareness. Very personal, whole-hearted methods, like those suggested in this book. Frustration, impermanence and the illusion of separateness is inevitable. Practicing methods of centering, especially amongst the difficult urges, invites us to calm the stressful and chaotic things that are happening inside and outside of us. The calmer we get on the inside, the more connected we are with our Spirit; as it is always leading us.

What we know about dieting.

When your mind is focused on aesthetically changing your body through altered food intake, you will eventually get what you want. Well, at least for a little while. Long-term dieting studies show that more than two-thirds of dieters regain more weight than they lost. Many studies have concluded that over restricting intake (food groups or food types) leads to more weight gained over time, even after accounting for genetics. The biochemical response is becoming more clear, and it's not just about willpower over food. [2]

If you eat, solely to change the aesthetics of your body, be prepared to challenge your relationship with food. Non-sustainable, fad diets and dictated food plans have a way of making you a slave to a "perfect" way of eating. Not everyone is cut out to micromanage their macronutrients, or are interested in buying prescribed foods and supplements for the duration of a plan. Most people can tolerate dictated meal plans for about six weeks. Dieters return to old patterns, reporting feelings of failure, shame, blame and guilt. Pounds rapidly return because there were no behavior changes that addressing prior habits. **I believe that diets and intuitive eating *skills* do not have to be mutually exclusive. Use them both!** Intuitive eating is a wonderful concept that I practice and encourage, but not without coupling it with optimal nutrition education. "Moderation" can look very different to a culturally diverse nation.

If you were my client, I'd want to discuss the dietary concepts you like, expose what we know about them, then *possibly* blend them. I think that blending certain foreign concepts (albeit ancient or classical) along with current research, education, mindfulness and common sense, make for awesome nutrition outcomes! Consult with your local registered dietitian. Visit **www.eatright.org/find_an_expert** for a nationwide professional directory.

Part 2: Body Image

How you see your body significantly influences your mental health. Body Image is defined as the subjective picture a person mentally creates of their physical appearance. This ideal or intellectual image of your body is influenced by cultural, societal, relational, and physical changes that happen in your lifetime.[3]

When I was in the depths of my eating disorder, I had a mis-measured body image. My self-image didn't include my personality characteristics and talents. My self-worth was summed up by two things: body shape and size. My body and I were in a bad relationship and I was always trying to break up with her; recreate her. In the beginning, I didn't realize that the way I was thinking about my body was affecting how I felt inside it. My quest for perfectionism was heavily influenced by the opinions and beliefs of others. I compared my body to other bodies- often ones that were unrealistic for my frame. It took a long time to appreciate my unique beauty in broader terms. I still struggle sometimes to see my body as an instrument instead of an ornament. I am now more equipped to filter information I receive through media outlets about the "ideal woman," especially those of my fitness profession.

I have girlfriends that have incredible positive body images. The kind of body image I admire in them is one that emphasizes perceived assets and understates perceived flaws. As my self-respect increases, so does my positive body image. Healthy minded men and women will agree, that a man or woman that owns their body shape (knowing it has no bearing on their value as a human being) is extremely sexy! If you don't believe me, ask! Now, if you don't believe them, then you may have just witnessed your body image wound talking.

According to the Center for Disease and Prevention, the average American woman today is between 5'3 and 5'4, 140-169 pounds. She wears a size 12-16 and has a waist circumference of 35-39 inches.[4] Thirty-six percent of American adults are obese. Whether you are below this average or within it, your weight isn't the only determent to your health. Studies are inconclusive, but is there health at every size, just as there is sickness at every size? [5] Using common sense, eating well, exercising, along with annual blood profiles completed by your doctor can usually determine if you're in good health.

Body image is subjective. If you think positively about the way your physical body looks, despite what media influencers consider ideal, you are pioneering a healthy body image movement. The research is staggering. Body image is culturally influenced, primarily by television, cinema, advertising, and social media. According to a survey conducted by Statistic Brain Research Institute in 2017, American women and girls are not at one with the size and shape of their bodies.[6] See chart on the following page.

Responses to Body Image Questions and Statistics on U.S. Weight Loss Industy

Percent of all women who are unhappy with their bodies and resort to dieting	91 %
Percent of women who say the images of women in the media makes them feel insecure	80 %
Percent of college-aged girls who feel pressured to be a certain weight	58 %
Percent of girls in 1st through 3rd grade who want to be thinner	42 %
Percent of 10-year old girls who are afraid of being fat	81 %
Percent of teenage girls who are, or think they should be, on a diet	53 %
Percent of teenage girls who reported being teased about their weight	30 %
Percent of teenage boys who reported being teased about their weight	25 %
Percent of 15-17-year-old girls who want to change at least one aspect of their physical appearance	90 %
Percent of teen boys using unproven supplements and/or steroids	12 %
Percent of girls age 15-17 who acknowledged having an eating disorder	13 %
Percent of women who stated they would consider cosmetic surgery in the future	40 %
Percent of men who stated they would consider cosmetic surgery in the future	20 %
Total annual revenue of the weight loss industry	$55,400,000,000
Total number of people with an eating disorder in the U.S.	8,000,000

It's not true that eating healthy *should* come from a desire to care for your body, and not change it. I know plenty of athletes who depend on changing their bodies to stay physically relevant in their sport (competitive jockey's, tandem surfers, ice skaters, bodybuilders and wrestlers, to name a few). They may be harming their long-term health, but they don't care. Their mind is focused on doing what it takes to excel at a sport they love. I'm not encouraging their lifestyle strategy, but I'm not judging it either! When that role expires, often times the debris of it will bring them to books like this one. I didn't write this book for athletes still active in this type of demanding sport. I wrote it for those that seek food and body liberation NOW!

When you walk by a mirror, what is your internal dialogue? How you speak to yourself when you look in the mirror, *matters!* As you seek to positively change your body image, the body will follow your mind and becomes enlivened! If you witness your mind thinking negative thoughts about your body, NOTICE you are in the grip of the ego, experiencing guilt or shame. These destructive emotions change our attitudes and cause us to focus on our mistakes or misdeeds. Practice speaking kindly to yourself. If you make a mistake and feel guilty about it, learn from it and move on. REMINDER! Everyone makes mistakes! You can't learn anything without making mistakes! But, please remember that shame creates blocks. You must not block! Find your positive body image voice, even if its meek, give it a bullhorn if you must. Then, slow down to hear it- listen to yourself.

Reality check! You DO NOT have to reshape your body or revamp your diet to feel good about yourself! Re-route your thinking, and your physical body will follow. The greatest love of your life is the person you see in the mirror; become aware of your inner dialogue with every glance.

Ⓢ Sweet Spot

Set a timer for three minutes. Go sit in front of a large mirror. One in which you can see your full body and get up close to your reflection. Get very close. Stare into your own eyes for as long as you can. Don't look away! Then, once the time goes off, take two to three steps back. Look at yourself as a whole. Don't focus on any one part of you. If it helps you to see the whole, focus back to your eyes. Witness your thoughts for as long as you can. Be gentle with yourself as you may witness you inner bully. When you notice negative thoughts, ask yourself, **"Who told me that?"** Close your intimate sesion by speaking this mantra aloud: **"You're the one I want."** Repeat it three times slowly.

Part 3: Gratitude

Eckhart Tolle reminds us, that "If the only prayer you ever say in your entire life is "Thank you," it will be enough." Merriam Webster defines the word gratitude as "that of being pleasing or being thankful." [7] To feel grateful is to feel thankful for something. There is synergy between gratitude, calmness and being grounded. When your nerves are calmed, you're far more effective in everything you do. Being grateful has the influence to shift your perspective in moments of anger, sadness, fear and confusion. In addition to rerouting brain activity to produce a happier state of being.

Here's how it works. When you choose to have an attitude of gratitude, you instantly redirect your focus from trouble and worry to surrender. Surrender is our voluntary release of the need to control. As you practice surrendering, peace enters, you become pregnant with positive vibes . In this way, anxiety is reduced, if not eliminated, and space is created around what is. Sometimes practicing gratitude provides a solution, a complete redirection of choice, and can sometimes freeze you in your tracks. Gratitude is the backbone of change itself.

The next time you are experiencing trouble or worry, try being grateful for what is occurring in that moment—especially if you're thinking, "NO, THIS SHOULD NOT BE HAPPENING!" I think this is the greatest challenge of all: Instead of repeating the depressive stories, or complaining, try uttering a "thank you" right in the middle of it.

Shame statements	Gratitude shift
"I want my comfort foods and I know I shouldn't eat them."	I am grateful I have memories of these foods in my childhood. I am grateful that I can fill myself up emotionally without the use of comfort food.
"My clothes do not fit anymore. I am out of control!"	I am grateful that I have enjoyed my life these past few weeks, months, etc. I am grateful for all the delicious foods I have nourished my body with lately.
"I know I should, but I don't want to exercise."	I am grateful that I am able to move my body. I am grateful that I am becoming healthier and stronger. I am grateful I am able to listen to my body when it is truly calling for rest.
"I don't want to meal prep. I don't want to make the time."	I am grateful to have food in my refrigerator to nourish my body. I am grateful for the use of my hands to prepare a nourishing meal for myself and others.

Ask yourself, **"How can I be more grateful?"** Start to see things in your life as a gift, not a hindrance. I best practice gratitude by writing, however, there are a few other practices that I believe are worth sharing. Here are five ways to help you find gratitude, almost immediately.

1. Keep a gratitude journal. Try writing down five good things about each day. Have you received good news, gifts, words of affirmation, grace, or experiences that bring you joy? Sit down for a few minutes to express gratitude. Recalling those favorite moments of your day, even if they're associated with ordinary things, can provide a snapshot reminder of the good things in your life, *right now!*

2. Meditation questions. Naikan is a Japanese meditation technique that involves reflecting on three distinct questions.[8]

> **These questions may provide a realistic view of our conduct.**
> 1.   "What have I received from _____?"
> 2.   "What have I given to _____?"
> 3.   "What troubles and difficulty have I caused?"

3. Speak prayers of gratitude. Spiritual prayers of gratitude recognize that what we have is enough. Prayers have the power to remove suffering, self pity and entitlement. To dwell on the good things in your life, and cherish what is present now, can change ordinary moments into blessings. One of my favorite prayers is simply, "Thank you, thank you, thank you." As soon as I say this holy mantra, I feel centered, *immediately.*

4. Come to your senses. Literally, come to your five senses! Get present! Touch, sight, smell, taste, and hearing are gateways of observance in having a human experience! You made the universal cut; you were born! Your whole life is a miracle, my friend. If you struggle to be grateful during times that are not pleasant, take a look around and start naming things you think are beautiful. Try to name as many things you see. For example, "my dog, Sadie Pearl, that tree, my table, this ring." A little gratitude everyday will bring you amazing results.

5. Be mindful of your words. By speaking words of gratitude over yourself and others, you are enforcing a language of giving, blessings, and abundance. SPEAK UP on how good OTHERS have been to you, instead of how good you've been to others. We transform the hearts of others with words of affirmation!

Part 4: Paying it Forward

Maya Angelo reminds us, *"When you learn, teach. When you get, give."* (Angelo, 2011)

To the people I have been able to serve, thank you, thank you, thank you! Many wonderful people asked me to write this book. They encouraged me, which made all the difference. If you were led to purchase this book, I believe it was of divine order. If you have worked its contents to this final phase, I bow to you.

My two closing requests: If you have been inspired or liberated as a result of this book, I invite you to share your experience with me. Whether it is short or lengthy, please email me directly! My contact information is in the prefix of this book. Secondly, I ask that you pay it forward. Please share a copy of this book with a friend or someone whom you feel would enjoy it. I believe that even long after its publication, whoever is reading this now, is as equally aligned in its creation as I am. My hope is that *Evolve Healthy* will end up in the right hands at the right time, thanks to you!

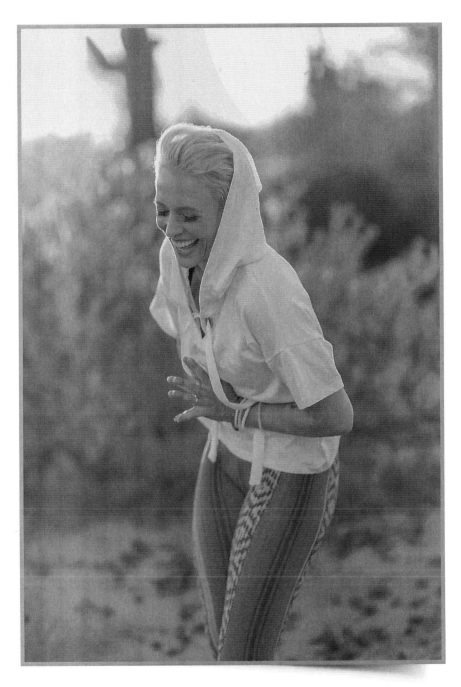

Thank you. Thank you. Thank you!

Jacquelin Danielle

About Jacquelin Danielle

Jacquelin Danielle, better known as Danielle, has a purpose to educate and empower food healing, movement and mindset with those that want to be helped. She walks the walk as a qualified healthcare professional, Registered Dietitian-Nutritionist, specializing in medical nutrition therapy and sports performance nutrition. Combining her dietetic profession with her national credentials as an NSCA Certified Strength and Conditioning Specialist, Titleist Performance Institute certified golf fitness specialist, and yoga teacher, sets her apart!

A graduate of the University of Alabama, Danielle has served in her field as an entrepreneur, visionary and leader since 2000. Her free spirit and passion for holistic healthcare has landed her leadership roles across the nation. Career highlights include: Outpatient nutrition clinic diabetes and lifestyle counceling (Pittsburgh, Pennsylvania), founder of Metamorphosis Fitness & Nutrition Studio (Clinton, New Jersey), Corporate Director of Health & Fitness at Foster Wheeler, Inc. (Clinton, New Jersey), Director of Fitness and Wellness at Enchantment Resort (Sedona, Arizona), fitness adventure retreat leader at Nemacolin Woodlands Resort (Farmington, Pennslyvania), founder of the first outpatient nutrition clinic in Etowah County (Gadsden, Alabama), strength and conditioning coach & sports dietitian at ACE Gymnastics (Gadsden, Alabama), health columnist for *The Gadsden Times,* Director of Health & Fitness at The Country Club at DC Ranch (Scottsdale, Arizona), and health writer for *Arizona Foothills Magazine* (Scottsdale, Arizona).

Danielle has been a seasoned athlete for most of her life. She competed in all around, artistic gymnastics from age four to eighteen. She fell in love with strength training at the age of sixteen and hasn't stopped training since. She has competed in Fitness America competitions, biathlons, cycling tours, and women's flat track roller derby.

Danielle currently lives in sunny, Phoenix, Arizona with her beloved (above) standard poodle, Sadie Pearl. Danielle's favorite mind-body practices include: meditation, prayer, walking, Yoga, Qigong, stand up paddle board, cycling, and strength training. She finds creative expression through writing, dancing, singing, guitar, painting, traveling, camping, and thrift store shopping.

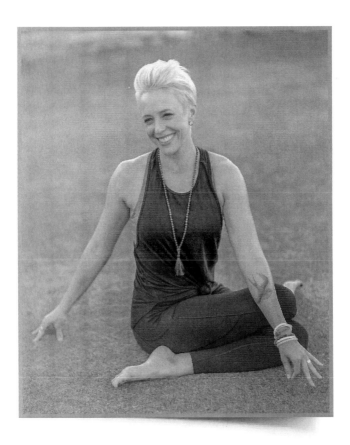

Acknowledgments

To my soul daughter, Sierra Rain Fryer. Your resilience, kindness, and healthy intuition inspires me. It has been a privilege watching you grow into a self sufficient, young woman. Don't ever forget you have everything you desire in life living inside you! Listen and trust your intuition! I love you, Cdog.

I humbly acknowledge my fierce, yet sweet spirited Mother, Norma Rippatoe. Mom, you fostered my entrepreneurial spirit, and showed me how to love complex people, and stand up for the underdog. Thank you for always providing me a safe place to ask the hard questions. I love you, Mom.

To my strong minded Father, Rick Ratliff. Dad, you encouraged my desire to learn, achieve and grow. You showed me how to create healthy boundaries. Thank you for being my teacher, and my friend. Mostly, thank you for doing *your* inner work! Your evolution has made a difference in mine. I love you, Daddy-O.

I wish to express deep affection to my siblings, Ryan and Jessica Ratliff. You are eternal extensions of my whole heart. Ryan, you taught me how to look beyond the status-quo (the ordinary), and how to lead. Jessica, you taught me how to play, create, forgive, and how to be a friend for life. I love you, Ryan. I love you, Jessi.

Dear April Jones, when I think of my life's blessings I count you twice. God has gifted us 27 years of loving connection! Ours is an infectious, enduring and empowering bond that inspires many. I cherish you as my sacred sister; my best friend of a lifetime! Thank you for your life giving support, encouragement, adventuring partnership, and conscious spiritual growth. I love you, Jonezy.

To one of my greatest teachers, Shane Fryer. We landed exactly where we needed for our soul's to evolve. Thank you for your love, beautiful laughter, the nomadic journey, and the spiritual lessons. I love you, Shane.

To my hippy soul sister, Kim Unhoch. Your high vibrations are 100% healing. You have positively impacted my life for the better! I adore our "just because" getaways to new places where only you and I would dare to explore, get completely lost, yet somehow find our way back with smiles on our faces. I love you, Kim.

Thank you, Zula Hill, Trull Hill, Tom Brown, Shannon Ratliff, Linda Fryer, and Janet Lankford-Moran, for drawing close and investing in our relationship! My life would not have been the same without your love's deposit. I love y'all.

To my sweet, curly headed canine companion, Sadie Pearl. Thank you for choosing me, walking with me, snuggling, for showing me kindness, devotion, and forgiveness every single moment we have together. SP, you make my heart dance. You're wooferful. I wuv you, sweet girl.

To my professional teachers and mentors: Thank you for your time, energy, resources, and believing in my gifts: Olivia Kendrick, Debbie Morrison, Mary Baun, Bobbie Sams, Richard Lively, Chris Bird, Robert Vance, Jill Clark, Kevin Johnson, Jessica Griggs, Michael Hawkins, Kristie Jaworovich, Katlyn Hatcher, and Kyle Draper.

To everyone that I did not list by name, albeiet an aunt, uncle, cousin, past friend, neighbor, client, student, boss, colleague, co-worker, or stranger--thank you for your love and support! And, for my nay-sayers, thank you too! Both energies have refined me. May we all simply SHINE OMMM!

References

1. Brene Brown. (2016, August). "When you deny the story, it owns you. When you own the story, you get to write the ending!" [Tweet]. Retrieved from https://twitter.com/BreneBrown/status/770254925494296577

2. Malcom, Lynn. (2014, June 30). "All in the Mind. What the Science says about Willpower." Retrieved from http://www.abc.net.au/radionational/programs/allinthemind/what-the-science-says-about-willpower/5560352

3. Charles, S., & Carstensen, L. L. (2010). "Social and Emotional Aging." Annual *Review of Psychology*, 61, 383–409. http://doi.org/10.1146/annurev.psych.093008.100448

4. Healthy Horns University Health Services. (2018, May) "Body Image" Retrieved from https://www.healthyhorns.utexas.edu/n_bodyimage.html

5. Penney, T. L., & Kirk, S. F. L. (2015). "The Health at Every Size Paradigm and Obesity: Missing Empirical Evidence May Help Push the Reframing Obesity Debate Forward" American Journal of Public Health, 105(5), e38–e42. http://doi.org/10.2105/AJPH.2015.302552

6. *Statistics Brain Research Institute.* (2017, February 17). Body Image Statistics. Retrieved from https://www.statisticbrain.com/body-image-statistics/

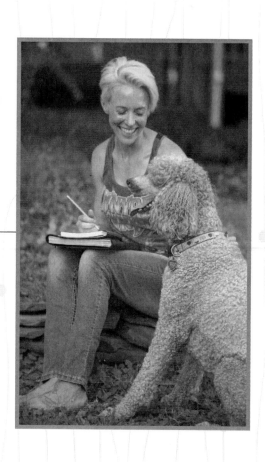

⟨ Index ⟩

In this section you will find the tools you need to complete this seven phased journey. There are fifteen Proactive Plan worksheets. Use one worksheet per week. There is a food group list (for referencing which foods belong to which group while food jounaling), and ten days worth of nutrition blueprints for journaling each meal in the *Evolve Healthy Food* Diary. For complamentary additional Proatic Plan worksheets and extra *Evolve Healthy Food* Diary worksheets, visit www.MindfulBodyRevolution.com

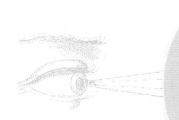

1. Proactive Plan Worksheets
2. Food Group List
3. *Evolve Healthy* **Recipes**
4. *Evolve Healthy* **Food Diary**

Proactive Plans

Complete one Proactive Plan each week. Write in pencil. Be flexible. Reschedule any broken committments within the same week if possible. *Refer to pages 32-41 for instructions.*

Here is an example a Proactive Plan:

My Proactive Plan

Week# _1_ of _12_   Dates: _11_ \ _3_ \ _19_ To: _11_ \ _10_ \ _19_

1. **Movement:** 150-360 total minutes per week
2. **Food Shop:** (1-2x per week)
3. **Meal Prep:** (1-2 hours per week)
4. **Mod Meal:** (1x per week)
5. **Self-care** (As often as possible!)

Monday
AM Strength Train 45min

P.M. walk dog 30min

Tuesday

P.M. walk dog 30 min.

Wednesday AM. Strength Train 45min.

P.M. walk dog 30min

Thursday
Self-Care = massage after work!

P.M. Walk dog 30min.

Friday
A.M. Strength Train 45min.

P.M. walk dog 30min

Saturday MOD MEAL! ☺   Self Care = Kayak Trip!!

P.M. walk dog 30min.

Sunday Food shop.
Meal Prep   Self Care = read under
P.M. walk dog 30min.   a tree at the park.

My Proactive Plan

Week# _____   Dates: __ \ __ \ __   To: __ \ __ \ __

1. **Movement**: 150-360 total minutes per week
2. **Food Shop**: (1-2x per week)
3. **Meal Prep**: (1-2 hours per week)
4. **Mod Meal**: (1x per week)
5. **Self-care**

Monday

Tuesday

Wednesday

Thursday

Friday

Saturday

Sunday

My Proactive Plan

Week# _____   Dates: __ \ __ \ __   To: __ \ __ \ __

1. **Movement**: 150-360 total minutes per week
2. **Food Shop**: (1-2x per week)
3. **Meal Prep**: (1-2 hours per week)
4. **Mod Meal**: (1x per week)
5. **Self-care**

Monday

Tuesday

Wednesday

Thursday

Friday

Saturday

Sunday

My Proactive Plan

Week# _____   Dates: _ \ _ \ _ To: _ \ _ \ _

1. **Movement**: 150-360 total minutes per week
2. **Food Shop**: (1-2x per week)
3. **Meal Prep**: (1-2 hours per week)
4. **Mod Meal**: (1x per week)
5. **Self-care**

Monday

Tuesday

Wednesday

Thursday

Friday

Saturday

Sunday

My Proactive Plan

Week# _____   Dates: __ \ __ \ __   To: __ \ __ \ __

1. **Movement:** 150-360 total minutes per week
2. **Food Shop:** (1-2x per week)
3. **Meal Prep:** (1-2 hours per week)
4. **Mod Meal:** (1x per week)
5. **Self-care**

Monday

Tuesday

Wednesday

Thursday

Friday

Saturday

Sunday

My Proactive Plan

Week# _____   Dates: __ \ __ \ __ To: __ \ __ \ __

1. **Movement**: 150-360 total minutes per week
2. **Food Shop**: (1-2x per week)
3. **Meal Prep**: (1-2 hours per week)
4. **Mod Meal**: (1x per week)
5. **Self-care**

Monday

Tuesday

Wednesday

Thursday

Friday

Saturday

Sunday

My Proactive Plan

Week# _____   Dates: __ \ __ \ __   To: __ \ __ \ __

1. **Movement**: 150-360 total minutes per week
2. **Food Shop**: (1-2x per week)
3. **Meal Prep**: (1-2 hours per week)
4. **Mod Meal**: (1x per week)
5. **Self-care**

Monday

Tuesday

Wednesday

Thursday

Friday

Saturday

Sunday

My Proactive Plan

Week# _____   Dates: __ \ __ \ __ To: __ \ __ \ __

1. **Movement**: 150-360 total minutes per week
2. **Food Shop**: (1-2x per week)
3. **Meal Prep**: (1-2 hours per week)
4. **Mod Meal**: (1x per week)
5. **Self-care**

Monday

Tuesday

Wednesday

Thursday

Friday

Saturday

Sunday

My Proactive Plan

Week# _____   Dates: __ \ __ \ __ To: __ \ __ \ __

1. **Movement**: 150-360 total minutes per week
2. **Food Shop**: (1-2x per week)
3. **Meal Prep**: (1-2 hours per week)
4. **Mod Meal**: (1x per week)
5. **Self-care**

Monday

Tuesday

Wednesday

Thursday

Friday

Saturday

Sunday

My Proactive Plan

Week# _____   Dates: __ \ __ \ __ To: __ \ __ \ __

1. **Movement**: 150-360 total minutes per week
2. **Food Shop**: (1-2x per week)
3. **Meal Prep**: (1-2 hours per week)
4. **Mod Meal**: (1x per week)
5. **Self-care**

Monday

Tuesday

Wednesday

Thursday

Friday

Saturday

Sunday

My Proactive Plan

Week# _____   Dates: __ \ __ \ __   To: __ \ __ \ __

1. **Movement**: 150-360 total minutes per week
2. **Food Shop**: (1-2x per week)
3. **Meal Prep**: (1-2 hours per week)
4. **Mod Meal**: (1x per week)
5. **Self-care**

Monday

Tuesday

Wednesday

Thursday

Friday

Saturday

Sunday

My Proactive Plan

Week# _____   Dates: __ \ __ \ __   To: __ \ __ \ __

1. **Movement**: 150-360 total minutes per week
2. **Food Shop**: (1-2x per week)
3. **Meal Prep**: (1-2 hours per week)
4. **Mod Meal**: (1x per week)
5. **Self-care**

Monday

Tuesday

Wednesday

Thursday

Friday

Saturday

Sunday

My Proactive Plan

Week# _____   Dates: __ \ __ \ __   To: __ \ __ \ __

1. **Movement:** 150-360 total minutes per week
2. **Food Shop:** (1-2x per week)
3. **Meal Prep:** (1-2 hours per week)
4. **Mod Meal:** (1x per week)
5. **Self-care**

Monday

Tuesday

Wednesday

Thursday

Friday

Saturday

Sunday

My Proactive Plan

Week# _____   Dates: __ \ __ \ __ To: __ \ __ \ __

1. **Movement**: 150-360 total minutes per week
2. **Food Shop**: (1-2x per week)
3. **Meal Prep**: (1-2 hours per week)
4. **Mod Meal**: (1x per week)
5. **Self-care**

Monday

Tuesday

Wednesday

Thursday

Friday

Saturday

Sunday

My Proactive Plan

Week# _____   Dates: __ \ __ \ __ To: __ \ __ \ __

1. **Movement:** 150-360 total minutes per week
2. **Food Shop:** (1-2x per week)
3. **Meal Prep:** (1-2 hours per week)
4. **Mod Meal:** (1x per week)
5. **Self-care**

Monday

Tuesday

Wednesday

Thursday

Friday

Saturday

Sunday

My Proactive Plan

Week# _____   Dates: _ \ _ \ _ To: _ \ _ \ _

1. **Movement**: 150-360 total minutes per week
2. **Food Shop**: (1-2x per week)
3. **Meal Prep**: (1-2 hours per week)
4. **Mod Meal**: (1x per week)
5. **Self-care**

Monday

Tuesday

Wednesday

Thursday

Friday

Saturday

Sunday

Food Group List

When documenting your food choices in the *Evolve Healthy* Food Diary, this food group list can help discern what foods go into which food groups. Not all of your dietary choices will be found on this list. It is not an exclusive list. It is meant to be a reference for your basic food choices. While enjoying combination foods, be sure to break down the food into multiple groups. If your food choice doesn't fit a food group (for example, a candy bar) simply write your food choice on the fillable lines below each plate diagram.

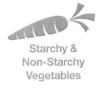

Starchy & Non-Starchy Vegetables

Fruits

Dairy

Whole Grains & Starches

Food Group List

This is neither an exclusive nor an exhaustive food list. It is intended to be a reference for correct food grouping while tracking food intake in the Evolve Healthy food diary.

Always review the Nutrition Facts on food labels for standard serving sizes. However, food label serving sizes may not always be the same sizes as indicated in this food group list. You may need to adjust the serving size on the food label to fit the serving size indicated below.

Protein

Animal-based protein sources include meat, fish, poultry, cheese and eggs. Anything that once had eyeballs, eggs and cheese is a protein source and does not contain carbohydrate. The more legs the animal had, the less heart healthy the source. Be mindful that animal fat is saturated fat. Know your portions! Too much saturated fat can cause heart disease.

Plant-based protein sources include beans, peas, lentils, nut butters and tofu. Beans, peas and lentils are also classified as a starchy vegetable. Their protein content is a high quality protein that offers carbohydrates and dietary fiber. Beans and peas may be categorized as either a protein or starchy vegetable food group. Nut butters contain more grams of healthy fat than protein grams per serving, therefore are categorized as a fat or a protein.

Supplements, such as whey protein isolate, soy and pea proteins are to be categorized within the protein food group.

RDN TIPS: Eat less red meat. Choose fish, poultry, eggs, and low fat dairy most of the time. Although the grams of protein is the same per ounce of meat, fish or poultry (7 grams per ounce), the amount of fat varies from 0-1 gram per ounce (fish, poultry) to 8 grams per ounce (red meat/prime cuts).

One serving is 3-6 ounces (3 oz looks like a deck of cards). If your body weight is <150 pounds, choose 3 ounces. If your body weight is >150 pounds, choose up to 6 ounces.

Meat:
- Beef: (select or choice grades, trim the fat), sirloin, flank, tenderloin, roast (rib, chuck, rump), steak (T-bone, cubed, porterhouse), lean ground round, top round, top sirloin
- Pork: Canadian bacon, tenderloin, center loin chop
- Lamb: Roast, chop, leg
- Veal: Lean chop, roast
- Venison: Back strap, tenderloin

Fish:
- (fresh, canned or frozen) cod, flounder, haddock, halibut, trout, tilapia, lobster, shrimp, snapper, tuna (canned in water), salmon, oysters, sardines

Poultry:
- Chicken: Breast, Cornish hen (white meat, no skin)
- Turkey: Breast (white meat, no skin), extra lean or lean ground turkey, domestic duck or goose (drained of fat, no skin)
- Eggs (limit to six egg yolks per week)

Protein Alternatives:

Tofu, whey, soy and pea protein powders. Twenty grams of protein powder is equivalent to consuming three ounces of protein from meat, fish or poultry. Generally, one scoop of protein powder provides twenty grams of protein. Check supplement facts for serving sizes.

Dairy

Animal-based dairy sources include milk, cheese, yogurt and kefir. These dairy sources contain carbohydrate, protein, and fat. The leaner the source, the more heart healthy the choice.

Plant-based dairy alternative sources include soy milk, nut milks, (almond, cashew) and rice milk. Nut milks are not a good source of protein. Nut milks contain more grams of healthy fat than carbohydrate or protein grams per serving, and is categorized as a fat or a dairy alternative. Rice milk is not a good source of calcium and is categorized as a grain or a dairy alternative. Soy milk is a good source of protein, but does not trump cow's milk.

Dietitian tips: Choose fat free, low-fat, and 1% dairy fat sources. Although the grams of carbohydrate is the same per serving of dairy (12 grams per serving), the amount of fat varies from 0-3 gram per serving (fat free/low-fat) to 5-8 grams per serving (2% and whole). Limit hard cheeses, but do enjoy them from time to time. This limitation is suggested due to their saturated fat content is high. This is not an exhausted list:

One serving is one cup (8 fluid ounces)

- Cottage cheese
- Ricotta cheese
- Milk
- Buttermilk
- Evaporated milk
- Yogurt (plain, Greek or conventional)
- Kefir
- Goat's milk
- Sour Cream
- Farmer's cheese

Fruit

The fruit food group include fresh, frozen, and dried fruits. Fruit offers a good source of dietary fiber. When choosing dried fruit, be cautious of added sugar. Check the ingredient list to determine if sugar is added. Citrus fruits, berries and melons are good sources of vitamin C. Fruit juices contain very little fiber.

Dietitian tips: Eat more fruit. It is the original fast food, portable, convenient, anti-cancer and nature's candy. Limit conventional fruit juices, because they lack dietary fiber. This is not an exhausted list:

One serving is 1 medium piece, 1 cup, 1/4 cup dried.

- Apple
- Applesauce
- Apricots
- Banana
- Blackberries
- Blueberries
- Cantaloupe
- Cherries
- Clementine
- Dates
- Figs
- Grapefruit
- Grapes
- Honeydew melon
- Kiwi
- Lemon
- Lime
- Nectarine
- Mango
- Orange
- Papaya
- Pumpkin
- Peach
- Pear
- Pineapple
- Plums
- Prunes
- Raisins
- Raspberries
- Strawberries
- Tangerine
- Watermelon

Non-starchy vegetables

The non-starchy vegetable food group includes fresh, frozen, canned and dried vegetables. Non-starchy vegetables contains small amounts of energy, and are loaded with micronutrients, water, and dietary fiber, they are considered a "free food group," because the goal is to eat more of them for better health!

Dietitian tips: Enjoy these foods on a daily basis. Try to consume 2-5 servings a day. Fresh and frozen vegetables have less added salt than canned varieties. Choose dark green and dark yellow vegetables, such as spinach, broccoli, romaine, carrots, chilies, and peppers. Broccoli, brussels sprouts, cauliflower, green peppers, spinach, and tomatoes are good sources of vitamin C.

One serving is 1/2 cup cooked, 1/2 cup juiced, 1 cup raw.

- Artichoke
- Asparagus
- Bell peppers
- Broccoli
- Brussels sprouts
- Cabbage
- Cauliflower
- Celery
- Collard greens
- Cucumber
- Eggplant
- Fennel bulb
- Heart of Palm
- Garlic
- Green beans*
- Kale
- Leeks
- Mushrooms
- Okra
- Onions
- Parsley
- Peppers (all varieties, especially red!)
- Salad greens (endive, lettuce, romaine, spinach)
- Sauerkraut
- Squash, summer and winter
- Swiss chard
- Tomatoes
- Turnip greens
- Water chestnuts
- Watercress
- Wax beans*
- Zucchini

*Exception to the list. All other beans are considered starchy vegetables.

Starchy vegetables

The starchy vegetable food group includes fresh, frozen, canned and dried vegetables. Starchy vegetables contain larger amounts of energy and are listed in a different food group to differentiate between non-starchy vegetables (a free food group), and starchy vegetables, where serving size matters.

Dietitian tips: Enjoy these foods on a daily basis! Try to consume 2-3 servings a day. Fresh and frozen vegetables have less added salt than canned varieties.

One serving is 1/2 cup cooked, 3 ounces
- Corn
- Peas
- Beans (pinto, black, white, butterbeans, kidneys, garbanzo, edamame, lentils, navy)
- Potatoes (baked potatoes, sweet potatoes, yams, red potatoes, new potatoes)

Whole Grain

The whole grain food group includes foods made with whole grains. Whole grains are a good source of carbohydrate, B vitamins, and dietary fiber.

Dietitian tips: Eat your whole grains! They keep your colon and heart healthy. Gluten free grains are listed below as a sub category of whole grains for those that are gluten intolerant. Of course, those that are NOT gluten intolerant may enjoy gluten free grains too. Gluten is a mixture of two proteins found in oats, wheat, rye and barley. These proteins are responsible for the elastic texture of dough.

One serving is 1/2 cup cooked, 1 slice, or 5-7 pieces.
If you weigh > 150 lbs, it is acceptable to double the portion listed, per meal to stay in energy balance.

Whole Grains

- Amaranth
- Barley
- Bulgar
- Cream of Wheat
- Couscous
- Teff
- Spelt

- Whole wheat pasta
- Oatmeal (plain, steel cut, old fashioned)
- Ezekiel bread (food for life brand)
- Ezekial tortillas
- Dave's Bread
- Millet
- Rye

Gluten Free Grains

- Brown rice
- Buckwheat
- GF pasta
- Quinoa
- GF cold cereal
- Grits
- Brown rice cakes
- Wild rice
- GF crackers

Fat

The fat food group includes three types of fat. Monounsaturated fat (most heart healthy), polyunsaturated fat (first runner up to monounsaturated), and saturated fat.

Dietitian tips: Do not be afraid to choose the fat food group. It is satiating! Accent your food with fats for awesome health benefits. Choose olive oil, coconut oil, and butter for dressings and cooking. Skip the other expeller oils and cream based dressings.

One serving one slice, one ounce, one teaspoon, or one tablespoon.
- Avocado
- Butter
- Cream (half & half)
- Raw Coconut & coconut oil
- Extra Virgin Olive Oil (EVOO)
- Hummus
- Natural nut butters* (peanut, cashew, almond, sunflower)
- Nuts (mixed, walnuts, peanuts, pecans, almonds, cashews, pistachios)
- Olives (black, green)
- Seeds (chia, sesame, sunflower, pumpkin)
- Tahini paste

Condiments, herbs and spices

Dietitian tips: Check ingredients for hidden sugars in condiments.

Below is a list of my favorite condiments.

- Balsamic vinegar
- Chili paste
- Chili powder
- Hot sauce
- Low sodium beef or chicken broth
- Mustard
- Salsa
- Lite soy sauce
- Black pepper
- Basil
- Cayenne pepper
- Chili pepper, dried

- Cinnamon, ground
- Cloves
- Coriander seeds
- Cumin seeds
- Dill weed, dried
- Ginger
- Mint
- Mustard seeds
- Oregano
- Peppermint leaves, fresh
- Rosemary
- Sage
- Thyme, ground
- Turmeric, ground

Combination foods

Combination foods are foods we eat mixed together in various combinations. Combination foods do not fit into any one food group. Often it is hard to tell what is in a casserole dish or prepared foods. Do your best to break down the food into the correct food groups. For example, frozen entrees and soups may include up to four different food groups. Document each food group into the *Evolve Healthy* food diary.

example:
Entrees (protein, dairy, grain, non-starchy vegetables, fat)
Soups (protein, non-starchy vegetable, starchy vegetable, grain, fat)

Document additional food choices that are not listed:

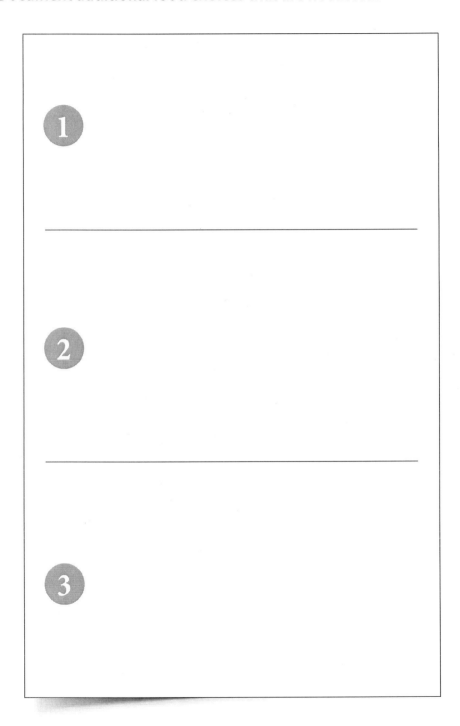

1

2

3

Evolve Healthy Recipes

Free Foods
Rutabaga "Pumpkin" Pie
Eggplant Tapenade
Garlic Greens
Clean Veggie Stock

Breakfast
Frozen Berry Parfait
Arroz con Leche (Rice with Milk)
Cornmeal Pancakes
French Toast
No Sugar Added Granola
Veggie Dream Cheese

Lunch
Clean Flatbread
Cindy's Basic Homemade Hummus
Clean Sticky Sushi Rice

Dinner
Slow Cooker Lentil Pilaf
Sauce of Whirrled Peas
Saag Tikka Masala
Ginger Sesame Marinade
Mashed Potatoes Plus
Clean Cheese Sauce

Dessert
Chocolate Hazelnut Mousse
Complete Banana Dream

© Jacquelin Danielle Recipes

FREE FOODS

Rutabaga "Pumpkin" Pie

Makes 8+ - servings of non-starchy vegetables.

Prep time: 30 minutes
Cook time: 25 minutes

Ingredients:

- 1 large rutabaga (wax turnip)
- 6-10 washed and scrubbed carrots
- 1 T pumpkin pie spice
- ½ t stevia powder
- ½ t sea salt

Preparation:

1. In a large pot, put 2 quarts of water on the stove on high heat and cover.
2. Peel the waxy coating off of your rutabaga and discard. You can do this with a knife or a good vegetable peeler.
3. Trim tops off of the carrots
4. Cut carrots and rutabaga into cubes no larger than an inch.
5. Once water is boiling, drop carrots and rutabaga in and cover until it reaches a boil. Simmer like you would potatoes for mashing, 15-20 minutes. Test for done-ness by testing that a fork passes easily into the center of the largest pieces of carrot and rutabaga.
6. When the carrots and rutabaga are cooked through, drain all but the last inch of the water into your sink.
7. Process rutabaga and carrots into a mashed puree (see methods in tips below) and add your stevia, sea salt, and pumpkin pie spice. If your preference is more pudding-like, you may wish to add more water.
8. Serve hot or cold with a dash of cinnamon across the top.

Tips:

A food processor, potato ricer, food mill or immersion blender is very helpful in achieving the smooth consistency that makes this non-starchy (NSV) dish such a treat.

Add one serving of medium firmness silken tofu to one serving and blend for a protein in addition to your non-starchy vegetable group.

This recipe scales VERY easily to large quantities, and it is great to have around when you feel like you need just a little something else to round out your meal.

Remember, you can always add more stevia, salt, and spice to taste, but you can't easily remove it.

This is a great extender for your single 3 oz. serving of cooked sweet potatoes.

Eggplant Tapenade

Makes 6 - 1/3 c servings of a free food - non-starchy vegetable

This recipe was inspired by ingredients--namely cheap eggplant on the sale rack at the local grocery store.

Prep time: 5 minutes
Cook time: 25 minutes

Ingredients:

- 1 large eggplant in fair shape, halved
- 1 T chopped garlic
- 1 minced red pepper
- ¼ c red wine vinegar
- ½ t sea salt

Preparation:

1. Preheat oven to 350*.
2. Spray a 9x9" cake pan with non-stick spray.
3. Salt generously eggplant halves and place skin-side-up in the cake pan.
4. Toss garlic and red pepper together and spread evenly around eggplant halves in the pan.
5. Cook for 25-30 minutes, adding ¼ c of water every 10 minutes.
6. When you can smell the garlic and eggplant, remove from the oven and let cool.
7. Puree eggplant, pepper vinegar and garlic in a food processor. Add salt and pepper to taste.

Tips:

Serve over pasta or on bread.

Add 1 T sesame butter (tahini) to a serving as a baba ghanouj spread.

Use as a vegetable dip.

Garlic Greens

Makes 6 -1 c servings of a free food

Dark, leafy greens contain loads of calcium and iron. The following recipe can be adapted to any season, fresh and frozen greens, and the end result even makes a great crustless quiche when combined with egg whites and cottage cheese.

Prep time: 10 minutes
Cook time: 10 minutes

Ingredients:

- 2 boxes of thawed frozen chopped spinach OR
  1 head of collards, kale, or turnip greens OR
  ½ bag of pre-washed collards or kale OR
  some combination thereof
- 1 onion, diced
- 1 t minced garlic
- 3/4 t salt

Preparation:

1. Heat large saucepan on medium and chop onion and garlic.
2. Spray pan with non-stick spray and add onion and salt. (Adding salt here helps the onions cook faster).
3. Rinse and chop greens roughly. For larger leaves like collards, a chiffonade cut can provide the ability to twirl your greens spaghetti-like on your fork.
4. Stir onion regularly. When it has started to brown, you may squeeze out the liquid from your frozen spinach, or add ⅓ c water. This will help deglaze the pan and cool down the temperature, which will keep you from turning your garlic bitter.
5. Add garlic and cook, stirring regularly, for 2-3 minutes.
6. Add greens and cook up to 8-12 minutes for fresh, 5-6 for frozen. Salt and pepper to taste.

Tips:

These greens can be a great filling for an omelet or addition to hummus.

Clean Veggie Stock

Makes 2 quarts of a free food

A good vegetable stock is a great base for a non-starchy vegetable soup, or a fantastic additive

Prep time: 20 minutes
Cook time: 60 minutes

Ingredients:

- 3 medium onions
- 4-5 stalks of celery
- 6 carrots
- 4 cloves of garlic
- 2 bay leaves

Preparation:

1. Heat a large pot on medium high on the stove.
2. Chop onions into a rough dice.
3. Spray pot with non-stick spray and add onions. Season liberally with salt and fresh pepper.
4. Clean and slice celery and then carrots no thicker than ¼"
5. And sliced celery and carrots to the onions, stirring occasionally.
6. Mince garlic and parsley and put those into the pot as well. Cook for 5 or so minutes, stirring frequently to prevent the garlic from burning.
7. Add 2 quarts of water, bay leaves, and simmer covered one hour.
8. Allow to cool and drain broth from vegetables, if desired.

Tips:

Omit salt if you intend on using this broth to soak beans, as salt will prevent beans from getting soft.

This broth can also be easily made in a crock pot overnight.

Freeze in ice cube trays once cooled for broth that is easily used as needed.

BREAKFAST

Frozen Berry Parfait

Makes 2 - servings of 1 fruit and 1 protein

This is a really satisfying high protein sweet snack with lots of antioxidants.

Prep time: 5 minutes
Cook time: 10 minutes

Ingredients:

- 2 c frozen whole blueberries
- 6 or 12 oz. medium silken tofu (6 oz. for women, 12 oz. for men)
- 1 ½ c Cheerios
- ½ c rolled oats
- ½ t cinnamon
- 1 tsp honey
- vanilla extract

Preparation:

1. Drain servings of tofu in a colander.
2. Preheat oven to 325* F.
3. Toss Cheerios and oats with cinnamon in a pie pan.
4. Shake the pan to distribute evenly and put in oven.
5. In a food processor, blend tofu and berries until combined.
6. Add vanilla and stevia to taste and blend until smooth and creamy. You may need to add a splash of water or skim milk to do this depending on how frozen your berries are.
7. Keep your nose and attuned to the oven, as you will start to smell cinnamon when your cereal mixture is a light golden brown (after about 10 minutes). Remove and allow parfait topping to cool.
8. Package into two flat sandwich containers and toss into the freezer.
9. Once they begin to set, you put half of the cooled topping mixture in each container and break it up/combine when you're ready to eat.

Arroz con Leche (Rice with Milk)

Makes 4 - ⅔ c servings of 1 whole grain, 1 dairy, 1 fruit

This is great served warm as either a breakfast food or a rice pudding type dessert.

Prep time: 5 minutes
Cook time: 20 minutes

Ingredients:

- 2 c cooked brown rice
- 1 c raisins
- 4 c skim milk
- ½ t cinnamon
- 1 t vanilla extract
- ¼ t salt
- 1 tsp. honey

Preparation:

1. In a medium saucepan, combine raisins, vanilla, cinnamon and milk over medium-high heat and simmer at a slow boil for five minutes to rehydrate and plump raisins.
2. Add rice and bring back to a simmer
3. Cook covered on low heat for 15 minutes, stirring more frequently as the mixture thickens.

Tips:

Microwave prep: This recipe can easily be made as single servings in the microwave and will maintain a firmer grain. Combine ½ c rice, 1 c milk, ¼ c dried fruit, and seasonings to taste. Cook at 60% power for 5 minutes.

Crock pot tip: In a small crock pot combine all ingredients except sweetener and cook on low overnight. In the morning, add honey to taste. If it tends to stick to the sides of the crock pot and gets too gooey, try the warm setting or reserve half of the rice to be added in the morning.

Cornmeal Pancakes

Makes 4 - 6" pancakes of 1 whole grain, 1 protein, 1 fat.

These cornmeal pancakes end up quite substantial, full of spinach and chiles and topped with broccoli and salsa. Loaded with veg, these cornmeal cakes are a savory meal and great anytime of the day.

Prep time: 15 minutes
Cook time: 15 minutes

Ingredients:

- 1 c liquid egg whites
- ¾ c corn meal
- 2 c frozen chopped spinach, thawed and drained
- 1 c mild green chiles, chopped
- ½ t salt
- ¼ t black pepper
- clean salsa
- 1 crown of broccoli, steamed

Preparation:

1. Combine chiles, spinach, corn meal, salt, pepper and egg whites and refrigerate overnight.
2. Heat 1 t EVOO in a medium nonstick skillet.
3. Pour ¼ of the batter in the middle of the skillet and cover, cooking until the egg starts to solidify in the middle, about 4 minutes.
4. Flip and cook another 2 minutes.
5. Top with broccoli and salsa.

French Toast

Makes 4 - servings of 1 whole grain, 1 3-oz. serving of protein

Prep time: 5 minutes
Cook time: 15 minutes

Ingredients:

- 2 c egg whites
- 8 servings of whole-grain bread
- 1 t cinnamon
- 1 T vanilla extract
- 1 tsp honey

Preparation:

1. Heat a non-stick skillet over medium-high heat.
2. In a gallon Ziploc bag, combine egg whites and cinnamon. If you are using bread that is two slices per serving, such as Alvarado St. Essential Flax Seed bread, add ⅛ c water in addition. You can add stevia before or after cooking according to personal preference.
3. Shake bag and put two pan-fuls worth of bread in to soak up egg whites.
4. Spray pan with nonstick spray and allow excess egg white to drip off of bread, placing them in the pan and putting in more bread in your egg white mixture. Putting all the bread at once in your "batter" will result in bread that falls apart, so get a good rhythm going with this.
5. Cook 3-5 minutes on the first side and flip when the egg whites in the middle have lost their clear, gooey appearance. Once you've flipped, cook another 2-3 minutes and allow to cool before packaging up.

Tips:

It's likely you will end up with excess egg white, in which case you should cook it up and divide evenly into 8 to make certain each serving of protein is complete.

This is only a half serving of protein for men, complete with an additional 3 oz of tofu, lean turkey or egg whites.

If you choose to use Raisin Ezekiel Bread, assume each slice contains 1 T of dried fruit for serving purposes and complete the serving with a scant amount of another fruit.

No Sugar Added Granola

Makes 10 - ¾ c servings of 1 fruit, 1 fat and 1 whole grain

This crunchy snack can be packaged up for an easy on-the-go snack. Unlike most granola recipes, this has no added sugar or honey.

Prep time: 15 minutes
Cook time: 60 minutes

Ingredients:

- 1 13-oz block of pitted baking dates (available in the middle eastern section) OR 2 c dried pitted dates
- 1 1/2 c unsweetened apple sauce
- ⅓ c dried raisins, apples, or currants
- 4 c rolled oats
- 3 c Cheerios
- ¾ c nuts (almonds, pepitas, peanuts, cashews, and walnuts are all great options)
- 1 T coconut oil

Preparation:

1. Finely chop dates.
2. In a small saucepan, combine dates and enough water to half-cover them--about 1 cup.
3. Heat over medium until mixture begins to boil, and then turn down to a simmer.
4. Add applesauce to small saucepan.
5. In a large mixing bowl, combine oats, dried fruit, Cheerios and nuts.
6. Remove date-applesauce mixture from heat, add oil, and allow to cool.
7. Preheat oven to 325* and line a baking sheet with parchment paper.
8. Add warm (not hot!) date-applesauce mixture to oats and nuts and toss with your hands. Add stevia, sea salt, and cinnamon or chocolate to taste if desired.
9. Once well-combined, spread out in a single layer on the cookie sheet and put in oven, tossing granola every 15 minutes.
10. Cook for an hour or so, until light golden brown. Crack the oven door and allow to cool overnight.

Tips:

If you love granola with milk as cereal, omit the nuts and oil.

Consider adding cinnamon or cocoa powder, flax or sesame seeds (fats).

Veggie Dream Cheese

Makes 7 - 4 T servings of 1 dairy

Veggies extend the usual 2 T serving of farmers' cheese. Check out the nutrition facts on whole wheat bagels and flat bagels--there are quite a few healthy options at your local supermarket. Alvarado Street makes clean bagels, too.

Prep time: 10 minutes
Cook time: 5 minutes

Ingredients:

- 1 package of farmer's cheese (7 servings)
- ½ stalk of celery
- 1 small carrot
- 1/3rd of a green pepper
- 2 green onions
- 2 chopped radishes
- 1 t salt

Preparation:

1. Finely mince carrot, celery, green pepper, and whites of the green onions.
2. Microwave for 90 seconds.
3. Mince finely the green of the green onions and radishes.
4. In a medium bowl, combine farmer's cheese, cooked veggies, minced green onions, radishes, and salt.

Tips:

You can also use spinach, chives and 1 clove of garlic to make another flavored savory cream cheese.

Use as a dressing for salad or serve over warm whole wheat pasta.

LUNCH

Clean Flatbread

Makes 5 - 7" chapattis of 1 whole grain, 1/5th of a fruit serving

This flatbread recipe uses fruit to provide the food for the yeast, which together with the steam created by the heavy pan will create puffy, tasty breads that

Prep time: 30 minutes plus rising time
Cook time: 25 minutes

Ingredients:
- 1 very ripe banana or 6 rehydrated dates
- 1 packet of yeast
- ½ c lukewarm water
- 1 ¼ c whole wheat flour
- ¼ t salt

Preparation:
1. Very finely chop and mash fruit in a medium mixing bowl.
2. Combine yeast and water with fruit and allow to proof in a warm spot for 5-10 minutes.
3. Combine salt, and ¼ c whole wheat flour on smooth, clean counter top. This will be your "bench" flour to prevent sticking when rolling out your flatbreads.
4. Stir ½ cup of the whole wheat flour into yeast mixture, then add remaining ½ cup and knead by hand.
5. Divide flour into 5 even balls and coat mixing bowl with butter before returning dough to the bowl.
6. Allow dough to rise, covered with a damp towel, in a warm place for 1-3 hours.
7. Heat heaviest skillet on high on stove and roll out dough into flat rounds, between ⅛" and ¼" thick, utilizing prepared bench flour.
8. Cook flatbreads one by one for approximately 4 minutes on the first side, flip when the bread begins to puff up and cook another minute or two on the opposite side.

Tips:

Top with 1 T peanut butter and up to 3/4 of a banana or other fruit serving.

When done cooking each flatbread, always allow skillet to heat back up with nothing in the pan for a minute or so to ensure a soft interior.

Basic Homemade Hummus

8 - ¼ c servings of 1 fat and 1 starchy vegetable

Cindy is a Yoga instructor at my studio. She battles rheumatoid arthritis and pushes through the discomfort a lot of the days to ensure better health. She has successfully been a part of the Mindful Clean Plate eating program after making up her mind that she was going to break her body weight plateau. Cindy and many others enjoy this simple clean hummus recipe.

Prep time: 10 minutes
Cook time: none

Ingredients:

- 1 16 oz. can chick peas (garbanzo beans)
- 1 clove of garlic
- 2 T tahini (a middle-eastern roasted sesame paste, found either in the ethnic foods section or alongside peanut butter)
- 2 T olive oil
- Juice of one medium lemon

Preparation:

1. Reserving the liquid, drain and rinse the chick peas.
2. Add chick peas, garlic, olive oil and tahini to a blender or food processor and blend until well combined.
3. Slowly add the drained bean liquid until the hummus takes on desired consistency (longer for smooth and creamy, blend shorter for a chunkier finish).

Tips:

This is a basic recipe and should be played with. You might like more or less garlic, tahini, lemon juice, olive oil, et cetera.

You can add things to this basic recipe such as roasted red peppers, garlic, parsley, cilantro, etc. Whatever tastes good to you can and should be added. Just be sure to keep your eye on the consistency when blending the ingredients. For example, I find when I added roasted red peppers; I need to add less of the bean liquid.

Adding non-starchy vegetables like clean artichoke hearts, spinach, roasted red peppers, and roasted eggplant will increase individual serving sizes to more than ¼ cup. No matter how much NSV you add, a serving will be 1/8th of the total batch.

Clean Sticky Sushi Rice

Makes 4 -2/3 c servings of 1 whole grain

This sticky rice can be used for sushi or rice balls, which can be easily discovered

Prep time: 5 minutes
Cook time: 45 minutes

Ingredients:

- 1 c rinsed short-grained brown sushi rice
- 3 c water
- ½ c rice vinegar
- ½ t sea salt

Preparation:

1. Combine rice and water in a saucepan and bring, covered, to a boil.
2. Once boiling, turn to a simmer and cook 35 minutes. Do not lift the lid at any point during cooking. You may swirl the rice in the pot early in the cooking process to reduce sticking.
3. As the rice cooks, combine vinegar, salt and set aside.
4. Set out a wooden cutting board or bowl for the rice.
5. When all water is absorbed, the rice is done. Dump it onto wooden surface and, using slicing and not stirring motions, drizzle rice vinegar mixture on the hot rice, allowing it to coat each grain. The mixture should clump together but not be wet (you may not use all of the seasoned rice vinegar).

Tips:

This rice is good for hand-rolls, rice balls, and maki (sushi rolls) with seaweed on the outside.

Utilize the rice before it cools entirely, as once refrigerated it is no longer suitable for making new sushi rolls or rice balls.

DINNER

Slow Cooker Lentil Pilaf

Makes 4 - 1 ¼ c servings of 1 starchy vegetable, 1 whole grain, and 1 fat.

Sometimes, packaged prepared foods can be a great inspiration for new meals. This is based on a ready-to-eat microwaveable healthy dinner I took backpacking with me. Enjoying this pilaf cold out of a freezer bag on top of a mountain is completely optional, but highly recommended.

Prep time: 20 minutes
Cook time: 60 minutes, then overnight

Ingredients:

- ½ c wheat berries
- ½ c hulled barley
- 1 c green lentils
- 2 cloves chopped garlic
- ½ c canned green chiles
- ¼ c onion
- 4 t EVOO
- 2 t crushed mint
- 2 t salt

Preparation:

1. In a crock pot combine wheat berries, garlic, chilies, onion, olive oil, mint, and 2 c water.
2. Cook on low for one hour.
3. Add barley and lentils, along with another 4 ¼ c of water.
4. Cook four hours to overnight on low. It's done when the barley, wheat berries and lentils are no longer crunchy.
5. Salt to taste.

Tips:

Toss as a dressing hot or cold over a salad of lettuce and tomatoes.

Sauce of Whirrled Peas

Makes 4 - ¾ c servings of 1 starchy vegetable, 1 dairy

This sauce can be used cold as a dressing or tossed with warm spaghetti pasta for a great dinner or lunch.

Prep time: 5 minutes
Cook time: 5 minutes

Ingredients:

- 2 c frozen peas
- 1 c chopped frozen spinach, drained
- 1 ½ c skim or 1% cottage cheese
- 1 c skim milk
- 2 cloves garlic
- salt and pepper to taste

Preparation:

1. Microwave frozen peas for 3 minutes on high.
2. In food processor, combine all ingredients and process until smooth.

Saag Tikka Masala

Makes 4 - ¾ c servings of 1 fat with options for additional two starchy veggie, protein, and dairy

Missing your favorite Indian food experience? Tikka masala ("with sauce") is a british-ized dish that is a mainstay in the UK, and spinach is a great go-to veggie in Indian food. The following recipe is an Indian-fusion simmer sauce, fit for peas, chickpeas, lean chicken, drained cubed extra firm tofu, and spinach. Get the spices listed in the recipe below freshest from an Indian grocer or the local health food store that sells spices on-demand and in bulk from big ol' jars.

Prep time: 25 minutes
Cook time: 40 minutes

Ingredients:

- up to 2 of the three following:
  Protein: 4 servings of lean chicken or 4 servings of extra firm tofu, cubed and drained
  Dairy: 2 c skim milk and 2 servings of non-fat half-and-half
  Starchy veggie: 2 c chickpeas and/or green peas
- 4 t EVOO
- 1 package chopped frozen spinach, thawed
- 1 large onion, chopped
- 4 large cloves of garlic
- 1 6 oz. can of tomato paste
- ½" fresh ginger root
- 6 cardamom pods
- 2 t turmeric
- 1 t whole coriander seeds
- ½ t red pepper flakes (optional)
- ½ t cinnamon
- ½ t salt

Preparation:

1. Heat EVOO in your favorite large non-stick skillet on medium-high.
2. Sautee onion, cardamom pods, turmeric, whole coriander seeds, cinnamon, dash of salt. A dash of garam masala would be good at this point too, but not necessary.
   Sautee until the coriander pods start to crackle/pop and onions become clearer.
3. If you are using protein in this meal, add to the pan and cook until tofu

is crusty, or until the chicken is cooked through.

4. Add chopped garlic and microplaned fresh ginger as well as pepper to taste.
5. Add dairy at this point (optional). If you are not using milk, then add 1 ½ c water.
6. Stir in ½ can of tomato paste and spinach.
7. Simmer another 5-10 minutes, adding a couple tablespoons of chopped fresh cilantro if you have it.

Tips:

Remember, the big flavor here comes from heating your turmeric and coriander seeds at the beginning with your onion and oil.

If you utilize oil but no protein, starchy vegetables, or dairy, you can have this over brown basmati rice (cooked with cardamom pods and a few strands of saffron).

If you use dairy and omit two servings of fat free half-and-half, you can use the Indian yogurt condiment raita as an accent for this dish. Raita very simply, is plain nonfat yogurt, cucumber, lemon juice, fresh tomato, and coriander seeds blitzed in the food processor.

Though the serving might not be huge, it's a deeply satisfying dinner or lunch option, and your house will smell divine.

Ginger Sesame Marinade

Makes 4 - ¼ c servings of 1 fat

This marinade can be used for chicken or fish, but is also great with mushrooms, bamboo shoots, and broccoli.

Prep time: 10 minutes

Ingredients:

- 1 T fresh microplaned ginger
- 2 t sesame oil
- 4 cloves microplaned garlic
- 3 chopped green onions
- ⅛ c clean soy sauce
- ⅛ c rice vinegar
- 2 t sesame seeds

Preparation:

1. Combine all ingredients except for sesame seeds in Ziploc baggie.
2. Add protein or veggies to be marinated.
3. Cook as desired, using sesame seeds as finishing accent.

Mashed Potatoes Plus

Makes 4 - ⅔ c servings of 1 starchy veggie

Non-starchy vegetables can be used to bulk up more limited food servings during meals, such as non-starchy vegetables or fat. This recipe takes a nod from the low-carb craze and utilizes pureed cauliflower in addition to mashed potatoes to make a more substantial serving size.

Prep time: 15 minutes
Cook time: 35 minutes

Ingredients:

- 12 oz. potatoes, scrubbed and cubed in ½" pieces
- 1 head of cauliflower, rinsed well.
- 2 t minced garlic
- 1 T fresh rosemary, chopped finely
- ½ t salt

Preparation:

1. Heat 3" of water in a large pot on the stove.
2. Break up cauliflower into bite-size stems.
3. When water is boiling, salt well and add the potatoes.
4. Cook potatoes until partially softened, then add the cauliflower and cook potatoes and cauliflower until soft, about 10 minutes longer.
5. Drain potatoes and cauliflower well.
6. Mash potatoes and cauliflower, adding in garlic and rosemary. Add salt and pepper to taste.

Tips:

While well-cooked cauliflower can be "mashed" in the food processor with rosemary and garlic, using the food processor with potatoes will create a gummy mess due to the starches involved.

Clean vegetable broth may be added for a less stiff mash.

For a smoother, creamy mash, use a potato ricer or process mixture through a mesh colander.

Cheese Sauce

Makes 3 - ½ c servings of 1 dairy, 1 fat, and trace whole grains

A simple roux is the basis for this cheese sauce, which can be used on non-starchy vegetables or over whole grain pasta

Prep time: 10 minutes
Cook time: 10 minutes

Ingredients:

- 4 t farmer's cheese
- 1 c skim milk
- 1 T EVOO
- 1 T whole wheat flour
- ½ t salt

Preparation:

1. In a small saucepan, combine oil, flour, and salt over medium heat.
2. Whisk oil and flour intermittently, allowing it to bubble for 2-3 minutes.
3. Add 1 c milk, whisking regularly to prevent lumps and ensure even cooking.
4. The sauce will begin to thicken and you can turn the heat down to a simmer. Add the farmer's cheese, cook for a few more minutes until the cheese is thoroughly combined.

Tips:
You can easily make a roux in the microwave, with good regular whisking to prevent lumps. Just start with your combined flour, oil, and salt. Microwave for 2 minutes, and then add milk ¼ cup at a time, microwaving 2 minutes, and repeating until done. Mix in farmer's cheese as usual.

Replace 2 T farmer's cheese with ½ c pureed nonfat cottage cheese for a different texture.

Add 1 T nutritional yeast to turn the white sauce into more of a cheddar sauce.

Mix in 4-5 T clean red sauce to make this into an Italian-style pink sauce.

Smaller-scale pasta shapes such as alphabets and acini di pepe work great to maximize quantity of noodles and space for sauce.

DESSERT

Chocolate Hazelnut Mousse

Makes 3 - ⅔ c servings of 1 fat, 1 protein

Tofu is the unexpected base for this protein-rich dessert.

Prep time: 5 minutes
Cook time: 5 minutes

Ingredients:

- 9 oz. medium silken tofu
- 4 T cocoa powder
- ⅓ c hazelnuts
- dash of salt
- 1 tsp honey

Preparation:

1. Drain tofu in wire colander.
2. In a food processor combine drained tofu, hazelnuts, cocoa powder, honey and salt.
3. Process until smooth and creamy. If cocoa is still powdery after 2-3 minutes, add water a teaspoon at a time until completely combined.
4. Refrigerate until served.

Tips:

Once frozen tofu loses its smooth, silky consistency, so always store it where it won't freeze in your fridge.

Instead of hazelnuts, you can use almonds as well.

Omit the nuts and fat altogether and instead add a few drops of mint, almond, orange or raspberry extract.

Use nut butters instead of whole nuts, 1 T per serving.

Complete Banana Dream

Makes 1 - ⅔ c servings of 1 fruit, 1 fat, 1 dairy

Frozen bananas in a food processor makes an ice cream analog that makes a great breakfast or snack.

Prep time: 5 minutes
Cook time: 5 minutes

Ingredients:

- 1 very ripe frozen banana
- 1/8 tsp powdered cardamom seeds or 1 pinch of whole tsp cardamom seeds. May substitute cinnamon for cardamom seeds.
- 3 T. non fat yogurt, soy-gurt, or non fat cottage cheese
- 1 tsp honey
- 2 T natural peanut butter (topping)

Preparation:

1. Blend all ingredients but peanut butter in a food processor or blender.
2. Add PB as a topping!
3. Enjoy!

Tips:

Omit cinnamon and cardamom in favor of 2 T of cocoa powder to get your chocolate fix.

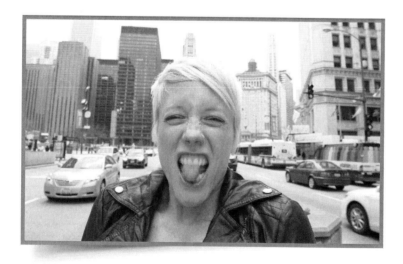

Add Your Favorite Recipes Below

(Food Diary)

The *Evolve Healthy* Food Diary's sole purpose is to empower food grouping, meal timing, and heightened awareness to food choices and emotions. For best results, document everything as you go. Remain judgement free as you unfold your eating habits and discover possibilities to create new ones. Refer to pages 61-71 and pages 85-86 for detailed instructions.

How to use The Evolve Healthy Food Diary:

How to use the

The **Evolve Healthy Food Diary**

Be sure to write date at the first meal of each new day

Document clock time at meal time

Circle each time you document a new meal

Date: __/__/__ Time: _____ AM / PM
Day: M T W Th Fri Sat Sun
Meal: 1 2 3 4 5 6 7

Date: __/__/__ Time: _____ AM / PM
Day: M T W Th Fri Sat Sun
Meal: 1 2 3 4 5 6 7

Circle each time you document a new meal

Check 1 droplet for every 8oz of water consumed at each meal + between meals

WATER

WATER

Choose your correct food grouping range. i.e. 2-3 food groups every meal.

① DAIRY — 4 oz cottage cheese

FAT

DAIRY

FAT

Free Food group

NOT Free Food Group

PROTEIN   VEGETABLE

STARCHY VEGETABLE

PROTEIN   VEGETABLE

STARCHY VEGETABLE

Check to acknowledge when documenting

WHOLE GRAIN   FRUIT

② 7 crackers   ③ 1 c. pineapple

WHOLE GRAIN   FRUIT

Space to document "junk food"

Close your eyes for a few seconds when asking yourself this question.

What am I feeling right now?
Love / Mad / Glad / Happy / Sad / Scared / Confused / Other

Where do I feel this inside my body?

What am I feeling right now?
Love / Mad / Glad / Happy / Sad / Scared / Confused / Other

Where do I feel this inside my body?

→ Space to document workout / movement

→ Space to document observations + celebrations

The **Evolve Healthy Food Diary**

Date: __/__/__   Time: _____ AM / PM

Day: M   T   W   Th   Fri   Sat   Sun

Meal: 1   2   3   4   5   6   7

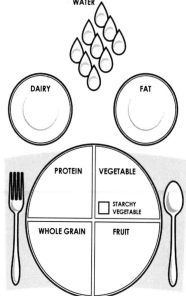

WATER

DAIRY   FAT

PROTEIN   VEGETABLE

STARCHY VEGETABLE

WHOLE GRAIN   FRUIT

What am I feeling right now?

Love / Mad / Glad / Happy / Sad / Scared / Confused / Other

Where do I feel this inside my body?

_____

_____

_____

_____

_____

_____

_____

_____

_____

_____

Date: __/__/__   Time: _____ AM / PM

Day: M   T   W   Th   Fri   Sat   Sun

Meal: 1   2   3   4   5   6   7

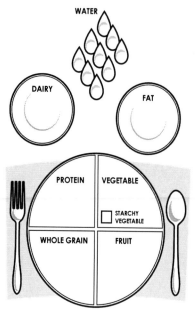

WATER

DAIRY   FAT

PROTEIN   VEGETABLE

STARCHY VEGETABLE

WHOLE GRAIN   FRUIT

What am I feeling right now?

Love / Mad / Glad / Happy / Sad / Scared / Confused / Other

Where do I feel this inside my body?

_____

_____

_____

_____

_____

_____

_____

_____

_____

_____

The **Evolve Healthy Food Diary**

Date: __/__/__   Time: _____ AM / PM
Day: M   T   W   Th   Fri   Sat   Sun
Meal: 1   2   3   4   5   6   7

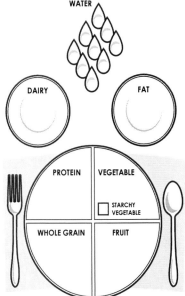

What am I feeling right now?
Love / Mad / Glad / Happy / Sad / Scared / Confused / Other

Where do I feel this inside my body?

_____

_____

_____

_____

_____

_____

_____

_____

_____

_____

Date: __/__/__   Time: _____ AM / PM
Day: M   T   W   Th   Fri   Sat   Sun
Meal: 1   2   3   4   5   6   7

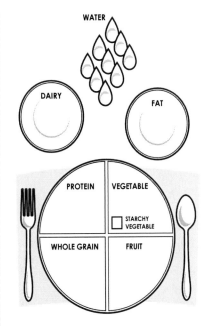

What am I feeling right now?
Love / Mad / Glad / Happy / Sad / Scared / Confused / Other

Where do I feel this inside my body?

_____

_____

_____

_____

_____

_____

_____

_____

_____

The **Evolve Healthy Food Diary**

Date: __/__/__   Time: _____ AM / PM
Day: M   T   W   Th   Fri   Sat   Sun
Meal: 1   2   3   4   5   6   7

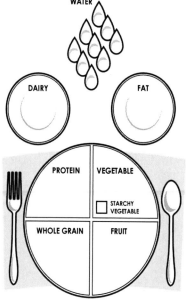

What am I feeling right now?

Love / Mad / Glad / Happy / Sad / Scared / Confused / Other

Where do I feel this inside my body?

_____
_____
_____
_____
_____
_____
_____
_____
_____

Date: __/__/__   Time: _____ AM / PM
Day: M   T   W   Th   Fri   Sat   Sun
Meal: 1   2   3   4   5   6   7

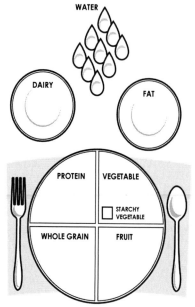

What am I feeling right now?

Love / Mad / Glad / Happy / Sad / Scared / Confused / Other

Where do I feel this inside my body?

_____
_____
_____
_____
_____
_____
_____
_____
_____

The **Evolve Healthy Food Diary**

Date: __/__/__   Time: _____ AM / PM
Day: M   T   W   Th   Fri   Sat   Sun
Meal: 1   2   3   4   5   6   7

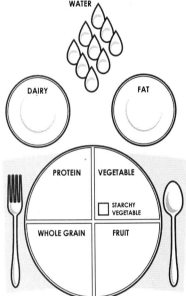

What am I feeling right now?

Love / Mad / Glad / Happy / Sad / Scared / Confused / Other

Where do I feel this inside my body?

_____
_____
_____
_____
_____
_____
_____
_____
_____

Date: __/__/__   Time: _____ AM / PM
Day: M   T   W   Th   Fri   Sat   Sun
Meal: 1   2   3   4   5   6   7

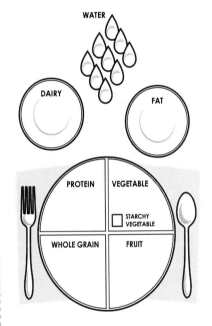

What am I feeling right now?

Love / Mad / Glad / Happy / Sad / Scared / Confused / Other

Where do I feel this inside my body?

_____
_____
_____
_____
_____
_____
_____
_____
_____

The **Evolve Healthy Food Diary**

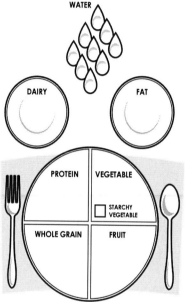

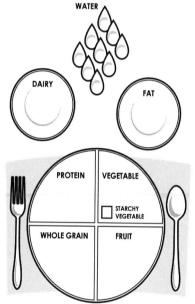

Date: __/__/__   Time: _____ AM / PM
Day: M   T   W   Th   Fri   Sat   Sun
Meal: 1   2   3   4   5   6   7

WATER

DAIRY   FAT

PROTEIN   VEGETABLE
STARCHY VEGETABLE
WHOLE GRAIN   FRUIT

What am I feeling right now?
Love / Mad / Glad / Happy / Sad / Scared / Confused / Other

Where do I feel this inside my body?

_____
_____
_____
_____
_____
_____
_____
_____
_____

Date: __/__/__   Time: _____ AM / PM
Day: M   T   W   Th   Fri   Sat   Sun
Meal: 1   2   3   4   5   6   7

WATER

DAIRY   FAT

PROTEIN   VEGETABLE
STARCHY VEGETABLE
WHOLE GRAIN   FRUIT

What am I feeling right now?
Love / Mad / Glad / Happy / Sad / Scared / Confused / Other

Where do I feel this inside my body?

_____
_____
_____
_____
_____
_____
_____
_____
_____

The **Evolve Healthy Food Diary**

Date: __/__/__   Time: _____ **AM / PM**
Day: M   T   W   Th   Fri   Sat   Sun
Meal: 1   2   3   4   5   6   7

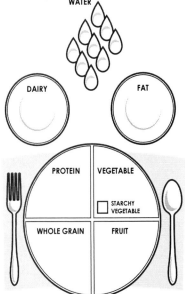

What am I feeling right now?
Love / Mad / Glad / Happy / Sad / Scared / Confused / Other

Where do I feel this inside my body?

_____

_____

_____

_____

_____

_____

_____

_____

_____

_____

Date: __/__/__   Time: _____ **AM / PM**
Day: M   T   W   Th   Fri   Sat   Sun
Meal: 1   2   3   4   5   6   7

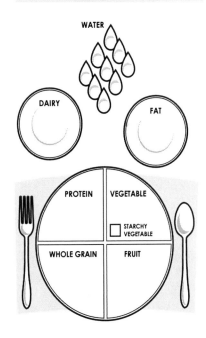

What am I feeling right now?
Love / Mad / Glad / Happy / Sad / Scared / Confused / Other

Where do I feel this inside my body?

_____

_____

_____

_____

_____

_____

_____

_____

_____

The **Evolve Healthy Food Diary**

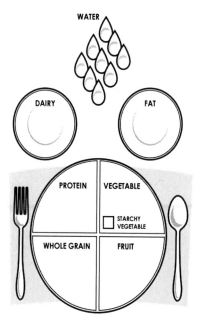

Date: __/__/__   Time: _____ AM / PM
Day: M   T   W   Th   Fri   Sat   Sun
Meal: 1   2   3   4   5   6   7

WATER

DAIRY   FAT

PROTEIN   VEGETABLE

STARCHY
VEGETABLE

WHOLE GRAIN   FRUIT

What am I feeling right now?

Love / Mad / Glad / Happy / Sad / Scared / Confused / Other

Where do I feel this inside my body?

_____
_____
_____
_____
_____
_____
_____
_____
_____

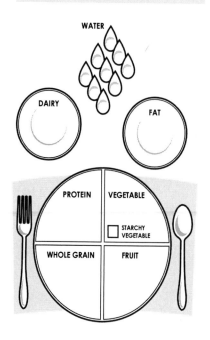

Date: __/__/__   Time: _____ AM / PM
Day: M   T   W   Th   Fri   Sat   Sun
Meal: 1   2   3   4   5   6   7

WATER

DAIRY   FAT

PROTEIN   VEGETABLE

STARCHY
VEGETABLE

WHOLE GRAIN   FRUIT

What am I feeling right now?

Love / Mad / Glad / Happy / Sad / Scared / Confused / Other

Where do I feel this inside my body?

_____
_____
_____
_____
_____
_____
_____
_____
_____

The **Evolve Healthy Food Diary**

Date: __/__/__   Time: _____ AM / PM
Day: M   T   W   Th   Fri   Sat   Sun
Meal: 1   2   3   4   5   6   7

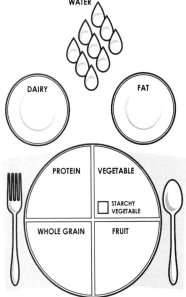

What am I feeling right now?

Love / Mad / Glad / Happy / Sad / Scared / Confused / Other

Where do I feel this inside my body?

_____
_____
_____
_____
_____
_____
_____
_____

Date: __/__/__   Time: _____ AM / PM
Day: M   T   W   Th   Fri   Sat   Sun
Meal: 1   2   3   4   5   6   7

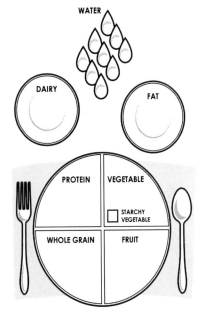

What am I feeling right now?

Love / Mad / Glad / Happy / Sad / Scared / Confused / Other

Where do I feel this inside my body?

_____
_____
_____
_____
_____
_____
_____
_____

The **Evolve Healthy Food Diary**

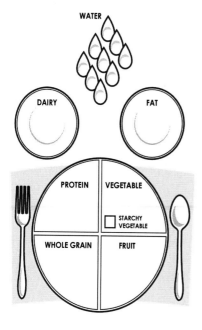

Date: __/__/__   Time: _____ AM / PM
Day: M   T   W   Th   Fri   Sat   Sun
Meal: 1   2   3   4   5   6   7

What am I feeling right now?

Love / Mad / Glad / Happy / Sad / Scared / Confused / Other

Where do I feel this inside my body?

_____
_____
_____
_____
_____
_____
_____
_____
_____
_____

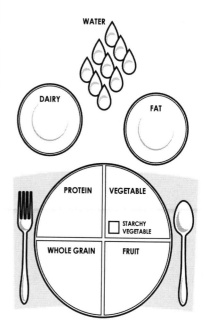

Date: __/__/__   Time: _____ AM / PM
Day: M   T   W   Th   Fri   Sat   Sun
Meal: 1   2   3   4   5   6   7

What am I feeling right now?

Love / Mad / Glad / Happy / Sad / Scared / Confused / Other

Where do I feel this inside my body?

_____
_____
_____
_____
_____
_____
_____
_____
_____
_____

The **Evolve Healthy Food Diary**

Date: __/__/__   Time: _____ AM / PM
Day: M   T   W   Th   Fri   Sat   Sun
Meal: 1   2   3   4   5   6   7

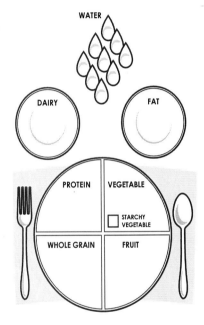

Date: __/__/__   Time: _____ AM / PM
Day: M   T   W   Th   Fri   Sat   Sun
Meal: 1   2   3   4   5   6   7

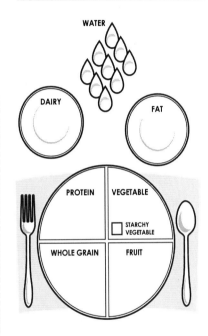

What am I feeling right now?

Love / Mad / Glad / Happy / Sad / Scared / Confused / Other

Where do I feel this inside my body?

_____
_____
_____
_____
_____
_____
_____
_____
_____

What am I feeling right now?

Love / Mad / Glad / Happy / Sad / Scared / Confused / Other

Where do I feel this inside my body?

_____
_____
_____
_____
_____
_____
_____
_____

The **Evolve Healthy Food Diary**

Date: __/__/__   Time: _____ AM / PM
Day: M   T   W   Th   Fri   Sat   Sun
Meal: 1   2   3   4   5   6   7

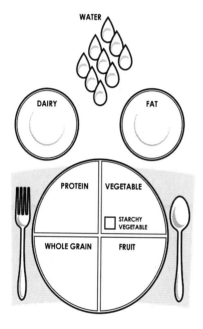

What am I feeling right now?

Love / Mad / Glad / Happy / Sad / Scared / Confused / Other

Where do I feel this inside my body?

_____
_____
_____
_____
_____
_____
_____
_____
_____

Date: __/__/__   Time: _____ AM / PM
Day: M   T   W   Th   Fri   Sat   Sun
Meal: 1   2   3   4   5   6   7

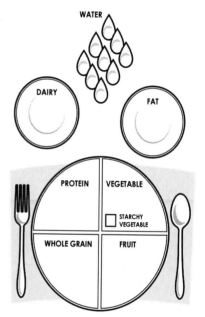

What am I feeling right now?

Love / Mad / Glad / Happy / Sad / Scared / Confused / Other

Where do I feel this inside my body?

_____
_____
_____
_____
_____
_____
_____
_____
_____

Evolve Healthy®

A Mindfulness Guide for Food & Body Liberation

Jacquelin Danielle, RDN, CSCS

Resources and Links

Contact Danielle for book signings, workshops, seminars, retreats and speaking events:

MindfulBodyRevolution.com

Social Media

Facebook: JacquelinDanielleRD
Instagram: JacquelinDanielle
LinkedIN: JacquelinDanielle
YouTube: JacquelinDanielle

River
Songbird
Publishing